try it!

MAKE-UP
TECHNIQUES

D0715411

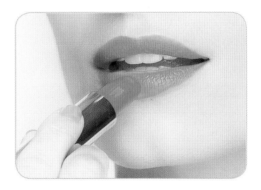

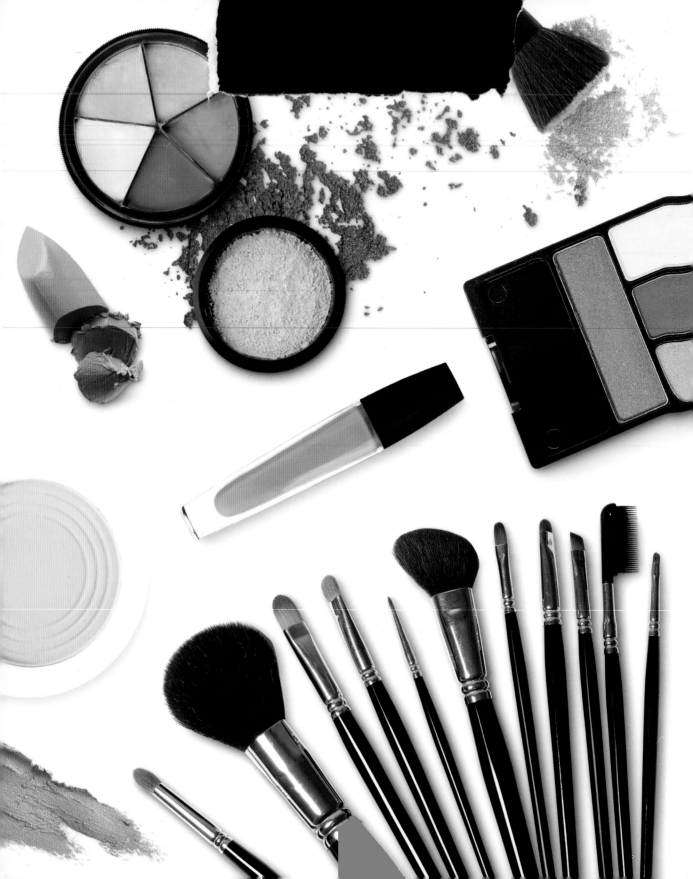

try it!

MAKE-UP
TECHNIQUES

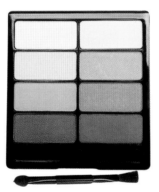

by Daniel Klingler

CONTENTS

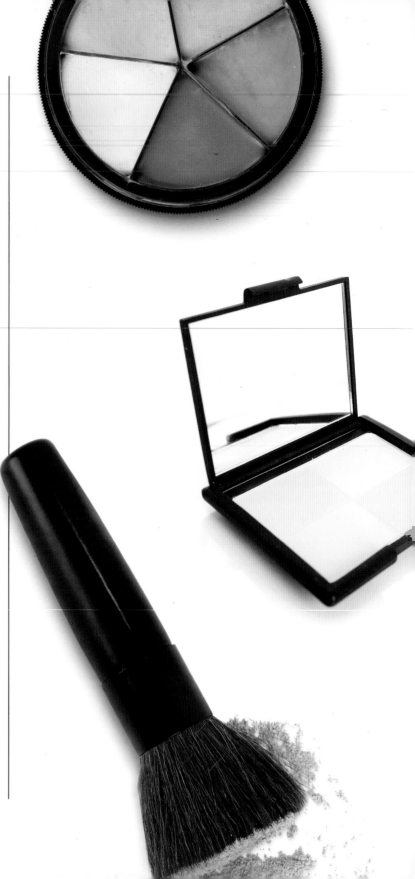

Penguin
Random
House

DK INDIA
Project Editor Arani Sinha
Senior Art Editor Ivy Roy
Art Editor Jomin Johny
Deputy Managing Editor Bushra Ahmed
Managing Art Editor Navidita Thapa
Pre-Production Manager Sunil Sharma
Senior DTP Designer Pushpak Tyagi
DTP Designers Nityanand Kumar and
Vijay Kandwal

DK UK
Project Editor Kathryn Meeker
Senior Art Editor Anne Fisher
Anglicizer Kate Berens
Managing Editor Stephanie Farrow
Managing Art Editor Christine Keilty
Jacket Designer Amy Keast
Producer, Pre-Production Andy Hilliard
Producer Stephanie McConnell

First published in Great Britain in 2016 by
Dorling Kindersley Limited,
80 Strand, London WC2R 0RL

Copyright © 2016 Dorling Kindersley Limited
A Penguin Random House Company
15 16 17 18 19 10 9 8 7 6 5 4 3 2 1
001 – 289126 – Jan/2016

All rights reserved.
No part of this publication may be reproduced,
stored in a retrieval system, or transmitted in any
form or by any means (electronic, mechanical,
photocopying, recording or otherwise), without
prior permission of the copyright owner.

A CIP catalogue record for this book
is available from the British Library.
ISBN 978-0-2412-4069-4

Printed and bound in China.

All images © Dorling Kindersley Limited
For further information see: www.dkimages.com

A WORLD OF IDEAS:
SEE ALL THERE IS TO KNOW

www.dk.com

INTRODUCTION

Have you ever looked at a make-up application in a book or magazine, or on the internet, and tried it out, only to find it wasn't successful? Are you overwhelmed by all the make-up options in the shops, to the point that you don't know where to start? In *Try It! Make-up Techniques*, I share all you need to know to create your best face, from choosing colours to fixing different make-up issues, and more. Whether your products and tools are high end or simply from your local chemist, the tips and secrets I share with you will allow you to create a beautiful look you'll be happy to show off.

This book follows the principles of art and design, meaning each make-up application is defined by the art principles of colour, shape, space, and form, and the design principles of harmony, balance, proportion, and emphasis. So while there are many ways you can do your make-up, I focus on the tools and information you need to create the most flattering look for yourself.

To start, you get a primer on what you need before applying make-up – from choosing and maintaining your make-up tools to prepping your skin. I've then broken down each feature by chapter, so you can zero in on its role in your make-up and what you need to make it look its best. I close with five classic make-up looks you can try. From a natural look to a metallic smoky eye, these looks have stood the test of time and are varied enough that you'll be sure to find one you like. You can then use what you've learned about your unique features to translate any look to your own face.

Whether you read the book cover to cover or use it as a reference guide, I hope it helps to simplify make-up for you. Please feel free to reach out to me at neckupdesign.com if you have questions about a product or application. Most importantly, remember it is not *make-up* that makes you beautiful; it is *you* that makes make-up beautiful!

PART 1
GETTING STARTED

CHAPTER 1

TOOLS

The correct tools are a must for creating beautiful everyday make-up looks. For example, I can't tell you how many times I have watched my clients use the disposable applicator included with their eye shadow. That applicator should be thrown away the minute the eye shadow is opened! So it is my personal mission to get a set of brushes, as well as proper disposables, into every woman's arsenal.

WHAT YOU NEED TO KNOW BEFORE BUYING BRUSHES

Walking through a beauty department can be very intimidating.

There are a hundred different brushes that can be used for make-up application, many of which can be very expensive. However, you can find each of these tools at different price points depending on your budget. Just remember the adage "You get what you pay for". Investing a little more money in quality will provide savings in the long run.

Beyond price, there are four things you should consider when investing in brushes: fibres, density, ferrule and handle.

FIBRES

Brushes are made from several types of fibre (bristles), which can be categorized as either synthetic or natural.

Synthetic fibres are animal free; this is what you'll get if you decide to purchase vegan brushes. Synthetic fibres are very soft, durable and easily cleaned. This makes them ideal for applying cream make-up. However, they tend not to hold colour pigments as well as natural fibre brushes.

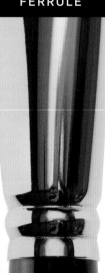

FIBRES

FERRULE

HANDLE

Natural fibres means animal hair. Goat hair is most commonly used to make less expensive natural fibre brushes and tends to be relatively coarse. You can find more expensive, often softer brushes made from squirrel, badger, horse, mink, and sable hair. Because natural bristles are more porous, they can be damaged easily when using cream make-up. Therefore, natural fibre brushes should only be used with powders.

DENSITY

Density refers to how many bristles are found in a brush head. Brushes that "dust" powder on the face, such as setting powder and blusher brushes, do not require as many bristles. Brushes designed to deposit more colour, such as kabuki and eye shadow brushes, should be denser.

FERRULE

The ferrule is the metal portion of the brush that holds the bristles in place. Nickel is the most durable metal for your brush heads, so stick with that.

HANDLE

Make-up brushes come with handles of different lengths and materials. Typically, a handle is either plastic or wood and either short or long. Shorter handles are best when applying make-up on yourself, while longer handles are desirable when applying make-up on others. When it comes to material, a handle should be durable enough to withstand pressure and balanced properly for comfort and manipulation.

Brush Head Shapes

The shape of the brush head is another potential consideration when it comes to make-up application. The following are some examples of different types and what they're best for:

- **Round, fluffy, flat synthetic brush head:** This is great for blending and buffing foundation into the skin.
- **Soft, round, large natural brush head:** This can be used for dusting powder on your face.
- **Soft, medium-sized, dome-shaped natural brush head:** With this shape, you can apply blusher and bronzer to the cheek area without disturbing your foundation.
- **Small, stiff, flat natural brush head:** This is ideal for applying eye shadows to the eyelid.
- **Flower-shaped, soft natural brush head:** The shape works to blend eye shadow on the lid. It is best used in circular motions.
- **Small-angled natural or synthetic brush head:** You can apply eyeliner and eyebrow colours with this type of brush. Use the natural head with powders and the synthetic head with cream make-up.
- **Small, flat, round-tipped synthetic brush head:** This is best used to apply cream lip colours.

FIVE MUST-HAVE BRUSHES

There are many more brushes you can buy to make your application flawless. However, these five brushes are the basic tools I recommend to achieve your overall look.

1 POWDER BRUSH

A powder brush is the largest of the brushes you need. It is used to apply loose powder, typically after foundation is applied. A powder brush can also double as a tool for blending make-up.

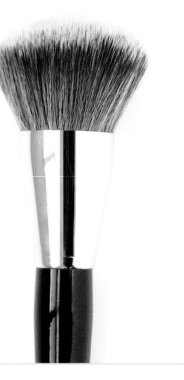

2 BLUSHER BRUSH

A blusher brush is a bit smaller than and not as full as a powder brush. Use the blusher brush to apply cheek colour powder (blusher or bronzer). You can also use this brush to apply contour colour.

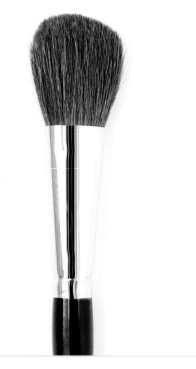

3 LARGE EYE SHADOW BRUSH

A large eye shadow brush, made of either natural or synthetic bristles, is great for applying lighter eye shadow pigments. I prefer a shadow brush with firm bristles, as I feel I have more control over the brush's placement and less drop-off (loose powder falling off the brush).

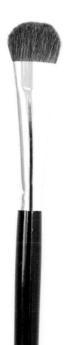

5 ANGLE BRUSH

This brush is my favourite tool. An angle brush is flat, cut at an angle, and comes with either synthetic or natural bristles. Use the angle brush primarily for eyebrow colour, or for applying powder and gel liner around the eye.

4 MEDIUM EYE SHADOW BRUSH (ALTERNATIVE: DOME EYE SHADOW BRUSH)

A medium eye shadow brush, made from either natural or synthetic bristles, is ideal for applying darker eye shadow pigments. Again, as a personal preference, I feel a firm bristle allows more control and distributes more shadow pigment; a brush with loose bristles does not hold as much powder.

An alternative to the flatter medium eye shadow brush, a dome shadow brush has dome- or round-shaped bristles that come to a point. The dome brush fits into the crease of the eye. The point deposits stronger colour into the crease, while the sides of the dome blend the colour on either side.

Why Two Shadow Brushes?

I include two shadow brushes because, if you don't clean your brushes regularly, it keeps the application less muddy. The larger brush is good for applying overall colour and a lighter shadow, while the smaller brush is good for more detail, and heavier, darker shadow.

OTHER BRUSHES YOU CAN USE

There are so many more brushes that assist in a flawless make-up application.

It's important to understand what each brush does. The following are some brushes beyond my five must-haves that you can also use to apply your make-up.

LIP BRUSH

This brush is typically synthetic due to the fact lip colours are cream-based. Its slanted edge can help you create a well-defined lip shape.

FOUNDATION BRUSH

A foundation brush is made from synthetic fibres and has a large head to help you cover more surface area on the face.

CONCEALER BRUSH

A concealer brush is made of synthetic fibres. Its small, thin size is perfect for applying concealer in smaller areas.

DUAL-FIBRE BRUSH

A dual-fibre brush is made with a mixture of animal and synthetic fibres. It's a great brush for blending powder, liquid, or cream make-up, giving an airbrushed look to your application.

BRONZER BRUSH

A bronzer brush is made from natural or synthetic fibres and has a dome-shaped head and dense bristles. As the name implies, it's used to apply powdered bronzer.

KABUKI (MINERAL POWDER) BRUSH

A kabuki (mineral powder) brush is typically short, with round or flat bristles. These bristles are dense to assist in applying a heavier amount of pigment.

ANGLED EYE SHADOW BRUSH

An angled eye shadow brush is perfect for applying colour into the crease of the eye, due to its contoured shape.

FINE-POINT EYELINER BRUSH

A fine-point eyeliner brush is made from synthetic fibres and sometimes comes in an angled ferrule. Its thin, pointed head is great for detail, making it useful for applying liquid and gel eyeliner.

SMUDGE BRUSH

A smudge brush can be made from either natural bristles or a sponge. This brush is designed to blend (smudge) a concentrated area, such as around the eye.

BLENDING BRUSH

A blending brush is made with natural or synthetic fibres, has a rounded head, and can sometimes be a little larger than a shadow brush. It's meant to blend shadow colours together, but you can also use it to add highlights to the cheekbones.

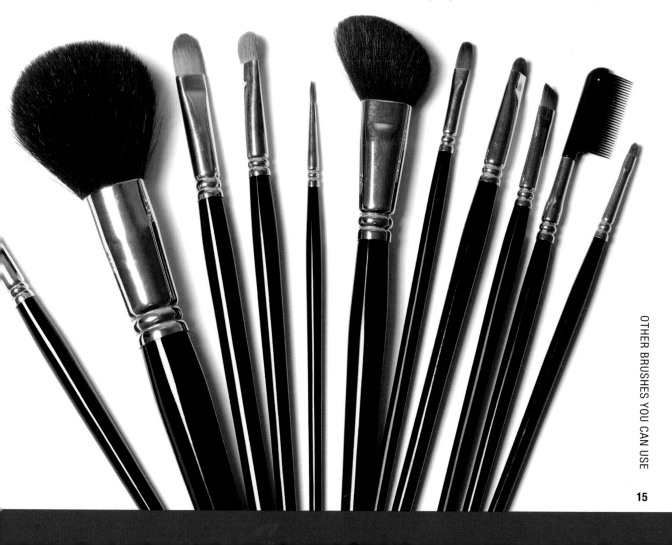

FAN BRUSH

A fan brush actually has several uses, including applying blusher, blending powders, cleaning up excess powder, and highlighting the cheekbones.

BROW BRUSH WITH COMB

A brow brush with comb is made with synthetic bristles and has a plastic or metal comb at one end. This tool is designed to brush and comb eyebrow hair.

The Best Tools of All... Your Fingers!

If you prefer not to invest in a foundation brush or concealer brush, your fingers will do the trick. You can use your ring finger to gently apply and blend concealer under the eye area.

Beauty Sponges

Another handy tool for your arsenal is the beauty sponge, a rounded applicator without edges that helps to distribute and blend make-up after application, without the appearance of lines. Think of it as the difference between a paint brush (streaks) and a roller (no lines).

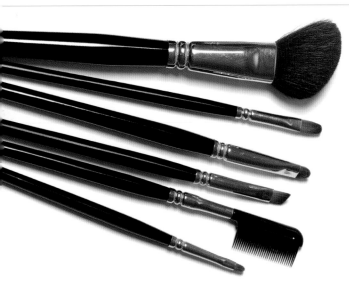

DISPOSABLES

To assist in your make-up application, I recommend using some disposable items along with your brushes.

These inexpensive disposable products can be found in most chemists. They work in a pinch, are hygienic, and keep your application neat and clean.

COTTON BUDS

Cotton buds are great multi-purpose tools when applying and correcting your make-up. You can use them to clean under the eyes where shadow or liner has smudged, clean around the lips, blend eye shadow, and apply lip gloss.

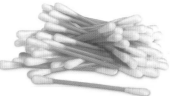

MASCARA WANDS

If you are in a family that shares make-up, you should invest in a box of disposable mascara wands. This will help you avoid any infections related to sharing the same wand for a product so close to your eyes.

MAKE-UP SPONGES

Make-up sponges, also called *wedges,* are typically made from latex. Use these sponges to apply and blend foundation, to apply concealer, and to clean edges around the eyes and lips after make-up application. You can even cut make-up sponges in half to reduce cost and waste.

BABY WIPES

I always have a package of baby wipes on hand. They're great tools to use during application, to clean any area where a mistake has occurred. In addition, baby wipes are a great alternative to more costly facial wipes. They may have soothing agents, such as aloe, and are available in fragrance-free, hypoallergenic versions for sensitive skin. What's good for a baby's tender skin is perfect for your face!

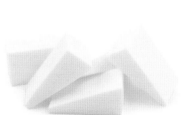

CHAPTER 2

SANITATION

Sanitation refers to the proper treatment of and disposal of tools. Over time, make-up products can become contaminated and harbour bacteria. Because your tools are moving between your products and your face, it's important to ensure that your make-up brushes, sponges, and other applicators – as well as your skin – are kept scrupulously clean.

MAKE-UP REMOVER

The last thing you want to do after a long day at work or night out on the town is take off your make-up.

However, leaving your make-up on can clog pores, cause spots and blackheads, and irritate the skin. It is very important to use a make-up remover prior to cleansing your face.

Make-up remover comes in three different types:

- **Make-up wipes:** Ideal for people who don't have the time (or patience!) for a lengthy cleansing regimen, these wipes are made of cloth dipped in facial cleanser. Once you've removed your make-up, you simply throw the wipe into the bin.

- **Oil-based cleansers:** Oil is an excellent ingredient to remove make-up, especially water-soluble products, because it dissolves the oil on your face without stripping away the natural oils your skin needs. Typically, oil-based products come in the form of creams and should be removed with cotton wool or a facecloth or flannel.

- **Water-based cleansers:** These cleansers remove make-up and tone the skin, returning it to its natural pH (4.5 to 5.5). They're a great choice for sensitive skin.

Creating Your Own Make-up Remover

Don't want to spend a lot of money on make-up remover? With a few inexpensive ingredients, you can create your own!

235ml (1 cup) water

2 tablespoons baby shampoo

2 tablespoons extra-virgin olive oil

Combine the water, baby shampoo and olive oil in a jar or container with a lid and shake; this will combine the oil and water. When you're ready to use the remover, apply it to a cotton wool pad and wipe your face.

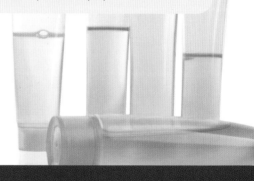

BRUSH CLEANER

Make-up brushes pick up dead skin cells, dirt, oil and product.

When you don't clean your brushes regularly, you are mixing this debris into your products and applying it to your face. Therefore, you must clean your make-up brushes regularly to keep them hygienic.

The following are tips for inexpensively cleaning and maintaining your brushes:

- In between uses, a baby wipe can help remove leftover make-up on brushes. I suggest using baby wipes that do not contain a lot of baby oil so you don't leave any residue on your brushes.

- Use washing up liquid and water to clean your synthetic brushes. Shake out any excess water and then leave them on a towel to dry.

- Because natural bristle brushes are similar to human hair, you can use shampoo and water to clean them. Once washed, shake out the excess water, form the bristles back to their original shape, and place the brushes on a towel to dry overnight.

Creating Your Own Brush Cleaner

Make-up brush cleaner can be expensive, so here's a way to make your own.

120ml (½ cup) washing up liquid

60ml (¼ cup) extra-virgin olive oil

Pour the washing up liquid and olive oil into a bowl. Swirl the brush in the mixture and rinse under warm water. Run the brush along your hand until the water runs clear. Shake out any excess water and place the brush on a towel to dry overnight.

MAINTAINING YOUR PENCILS AND PENCIL SHARPENER

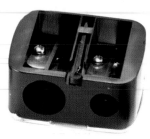

Your lips and eyes can harbour debris and dead skin.

Therefore, always sharpen your cosmetic pencils after every use, and be certain to replace the lid in order to keep your pencils clean.

Pencil sharpeners often come with a container to catch shavings. They are inexpensive and should be replaced once a year. However, you should still be sure to clean your pencil sharpener after you use it. To do this, empty the shavings from the sharpener's inner compartment. Next, dip a cotton bud in isopropyl alcohol (surgical spirit) and work your way around the inside of the compartment, as well as the blade. The alcohol acts as a disinfectant. (You may want to use a toothbrush to remove any cream left behind by the pencils.)

Using the Correct Pencil Sharpener

Don't use a graphite pencil sharpener (used for HB pencils) on cosmetic pencils. They are not nearly as effective, plus any cross-contamination from regular pencils can lead to you getting wood shavings and graphite in your eyes. You can find sharpeners specially designed for cosmetic pencils in the make-up section of your local chemist.

GETTING RID OF DISPOSABLE APPLICATORS

Cotton buds, tissues, wooden spatulas, and cotton wool pads are examples of disposable applicators. All are great tools for helping you achieve your make-up look (or removing make-up) and don't require any special cleaning before or after. However, disposable applicators are not meant for repeated use. They should be discarded on finishing your make-up application.

USE-BY DATES

I am required, as a make-up artist, to invest in a vast assortment of cosmetics. So you can probably imagine the internal conflict I go through when I decide to dispose of it.

Needless to say, all make-up comes with an expiry date. Your products contain preservatives that keep them from deteriorating. Eventually, the products will begin to break down and can become contaminated.

Most cosmetic products contain a suggested use-by date. If you aren't sure when to get rid of your product, look for the universal product expiry label on it. You should find a number indicating the length of time a product can be used (for example, 12m for 12 months).

That label aside, for safety and hygiene purposes, the following are the generally recommended disposal dates for your make-up:

- **Mascara:** 2 to 3 months

- **Foundation:** 6 to 12 months

- **Eye shadow:** 12 to 18 months

- **Lipstick:** 12 to 18 months

- **Lip/eye pencil:** 18 to 24 months

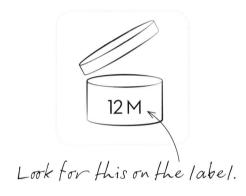

Look for this on the label.

Sharing Make-up

Be wary about hygiene if you share or swap make-up. Mascara and liquid eyeliners should not be shared, but most cosmetics can be disinfected by wiping them with a cotton pad soaked in surgical spirit.

CHAPTER 3

SKIN CARE

Your face is the canvas for a beautiful make-up application. Therefore, in order to have people avoid painting on a dirty canvas, I always start my make-up consultations with a discussion about good skin care.

SKIN TYPES

The first step to revealing your beauty through make-up application is good skin care.

To begin, you must determine your skin type to find the products best suited for you. Skin is generally classified into one of five categories: normal, oily, dry, combination, and sensitive.

OILY SKIN

Oily skin can change depending on the time of year or weather. It is caused or made worse by stress, hormones and/or exposure to heat or humidity. Other characteristics of oily skin are the following:

- Overactive sebaceous (oil) glands
- Dull or shiny skin
- Appearance of excessive blackheads, spots and blemishes

NORMAL SKIN

Normal skin is the least problematic type of skin; it's not too dry and not too oily. Other characteristics of normal skin include the following:

- No or few imperfections
- No severe sensitivity
- Barely visible pores
- A radiant complexion

DRY SKIN

Dry skin can crack and peel, or become itchy, irritated, or inflamed. If your skin is excessively dry, it can become rough and scaly, especially on the backs of your hands, your arms and legs. Other characteristics of dry skin include the following:

- Almost invisible pores
- A dull, rough complexion
- Red patches
- Less elasticity
- More visible lines

COMBINATION SKIN

Combination skin can be dry or normal in some areas and oily in others, such as the T-zone (nose, forehead, and chin). You will therefore need multiple products to address these different areas. Other characteristics of combination skin include the following:

- Overly dilated pores
- Blackheads
- Shiny skin

SENSITIVE SKIN

Skin can become sensitive for a variety of reasons. Most likely, it is caused by a cosmetic product, food or your environment. You can attempt to eliminate products that cause sensitivity through trial and error. Otherwise, I encourage you to consult a dermatologist to diagnose the sensitivity. Other characteristics of sensitive skin include the following:

- Redness
- Itching
- Burning
- Dryness

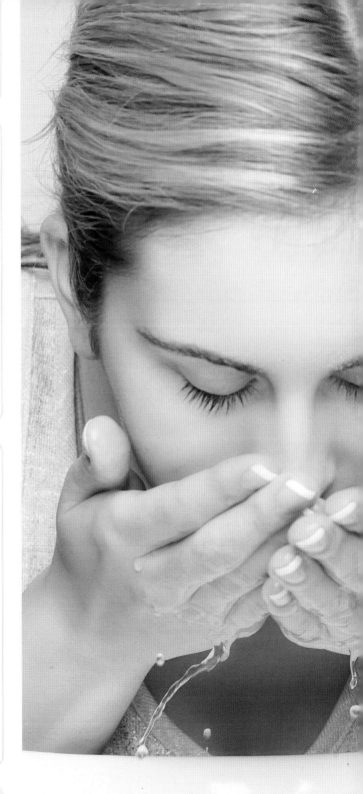

TEN POWER FOODS FOR HEALTHY SKIN

Diet is a large factor in the health of your skin.

As the saying goes, "you are what you eat". So before I get into skin care products, let's go over the 10 power foods that aid in skin health:

- **Cocoa powder:** This contains antioxidants that provide hydration. The caffeine in cocoa powder also benefits circulation in the skin.

- **Coffee:** You will find caffeine as an ingredient in many eye creams due to its anti-inflammatory effects. In the same way, drinking a cup of caffeinated coffee can help reduce skin swelling and inflammation.

- **Fish:** Fish contain omega-3 fatty acids, which reduce inflammation. This makes fish a great diet staple for those with acne-prone skin.

- **Fruits:** Power fruits such as blueberries, oranges, and strawberries contain vitamin C, a super-antioxidant. Vitamin C boosts the immune system, creates radiant skin, and helps blemishes heal properly.

- **Nuts:** Nuts contain protein, omega-3 and -6, vitamin E, calcium, and magnesium, all of which are good for fighting ageing.

- **Olive oil:** Free radicals can lead to a loss of two things in your skin that keep you looking young: collagen and elastin. Olive oil has antioxidant polyphenols that help defend against these damaging free radicals.

- **Peppers:** The antioxidants in yellow and orange peppers help decrease skin's sensitivity to the sun, meaning fewer wrinkles!

- **Sweet potatoes:** These contain vitamin C, which smoothes wrinkles by stimulating the production of collagen.

- **Tomatoes:** These are full of lycopene, a chemical that helps eliminate skin-ageing free radicals caused by ultra-violet rays. Eating tomatoes can also help protect against sun damage.

- **Water:** Don't forget about H_2O! Six to eight glasses of water a day rejuvenate cell growth, making your skin look plumper and more hydrated.

CLEANSERS

Cleansers are essential for removing dirt and make-up so you have a fresh palette to work with.

It is recommended that you only wash your face twice daily – any more than that, and you will strip your skin of its essential oils. Because there are so many types of cleanser, I find it best to narrow down your choices by choosing one based on your skin type.

Normal: You can use most cleansers on this skin type. Specifically, cleansers that lather with water and cleansers without alcohol work best. Cleansers with alcohol can dry out your skin.

Oily: Cleansers that are water-based are great for oily skin. Look for cleansers that contain some type of acid, such as salicylic. This acid gently removes oil and reduces oil production.

Dry: Cleansers containing moisturizers are ideal for dry skin types. Avoid using cleansers that contain alcohol, as they can dry out your skin further.

Combination: The key to cleansing combination skin is to identify cleansers that address the different problem areas. Foaming cleansers that are pH-balanced help correct combination skin. Avoid using harsh cleansers that may inflame areas of the skin.

Sensitive: Sensitive skin types can have difficulty tolerating cleansers due to the acids and strong detergents in them. Therefore, look for cleansers that are fragrance and preservative free. As with combination skin, you want products that balance the skin's pH level.

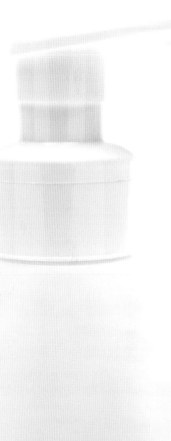

Acne Cleansers

If you have acne-prone skin, look for cleansers that contain salicylic acid, which is a beta hydroxy acid used to treat acne. Cleansers specific to treating acne will be clearly marked that they help with acne-prone skin. Agents in these products assist in topical removal of bacteria and dirt and the cleaning of overactive sebaceous (oil) glands.

EXFOLIANTS

Exfoliants are designed to remove dead cells from the surface of your skin. There are two types of exfoliant: mechanical and chemical.

Mechanical exfoliants contain abrasives such as microbeads, ground seeds, sugar, and salt. Almost any skin type can use a mechanical exfoliant. However, if you have sensitive skin, you may find this type of exfoliant to be too abrasive.

Chemical exfoliants contain a low concentration of "safe-to-use" acids. Chemical exfoliation is great for all skin types, but especially for those suffering with acne. This is because the acids used in chemical exfoliants go deeper into the skin, helping to unclog pores and reduce sebum (oil) production.

Caution!

I strongly encourage you not to use exfoliants with microbeads on your face. One reason is they may cause small abrasions (cuts) on your skin. Another argument against microbeads is that they are bad for the environment. If the product is not organic, the microbeads may be made from plastics, which can't be filtered during water treatment and will therefore end up back in our lakes and oceans.

Lip Exfoliation

Did you know your lips also benefit from exfoliation? Removing debris and dead skin allows your lip products to adhere better and keeps lips looking healthy. One way to exfoliate your lips is with a soft or baby toothbrush. Another option is to use a lip scrub, which you can find in any skin care aisle. Whatever you use, follow your exfoliation with a hydrating lip balm.

TONERS

I am going to be honest with you. For a long time, I had no idea what a toner was or why I should use this product. Therefore, I'd like to share what I've learned with you, so you know how important it is to use toner on your skin

Cleansers and exfoliants generally have an acid included as an ingredient. Acids (such as lactic or salicylic acid) are approved ingredients to gently remove dead skin, reduce oil, and unclog your pores. However, these acids change the pH of the skin, which is typically between 4.5 and 5.5, as marked on the following scale.

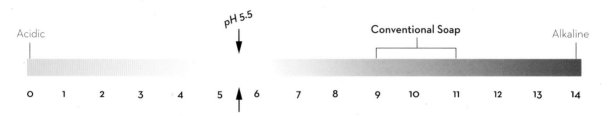

Acidic					pH 5.5				Conventional Soap				Alkaline
0	1	2	3	4	5	6	7	8	9	10	11	12	13	14

To leave the skin at a lower pH would cause the skin to become dry. A toner is pH balanced to return skin to its proper pH level. Additionally, toners remove excess debris and reduce pore size.

Toner can be applied either as a spray mist or by using a cotton wool pad. I recommend applying toner after cleansing and exfoliation and before applying serums and moisturizers.

EYE CREAMS

Eye creams are used to reduce swelling, dark circles, and wrinkles.

The under-eye area contains thinner skin and does not produce the sebum needed to keep the area moist. Therefore, it can be helpful to invest in an eye cream appropriate to your needs. As you mature, collagen (a protein that gives the skin structure, firmness, and elasticity) begins to break down. Eye creams contain ingredients such as retinol to replace collagen and reduce the signs of ageing.

The most common problems eye cream is used to combat are dark circles, puffiness, and fine lines and wrinkles. The following addresses the ingredients you should look for in an eye cream to treat those issues.

Dark circles: Contributors to dark circles include genetics, fatigue, broken capillaries, allergies, poor nutrition, age, and sun exposure. While a change of diet and lifestyle may still be the best way to combat or reduce dark circles in the long run, an eye cream that contains brightening agents like vitamin C, licorice, kojic acid, and niacinamide can help counter excess pigmentation and help stop the oxidation process that occurs on the surface of the skin. Retinols, peptides, and ceramides also work by thickening and strengthening the skin, making broken capillaries appear less visible.

Puffiness: While consuming salty foods and alcohol are the main reasons for puffiness under the eye, another way to combat this issue is to use an eye cream that contains caffeine. Most experts believe that caffeine stimulates circulation and constricts the blood vessels under the skin, diminishing the look of puffy eyes. As an antioxidant, it also protects the skin from sun damage.

Fine lines and wrinkles: If fine lines and wrinkles are your main concern, look for an eye cream that contains retinol, a powerful antioxidant embraced by dermatologists for its ability to smooth lines and wrinkles. As well as assisting in the production of healthy skin cells, retinol works by hampering the breakdown of collagen (which provides the skin's elasticity).

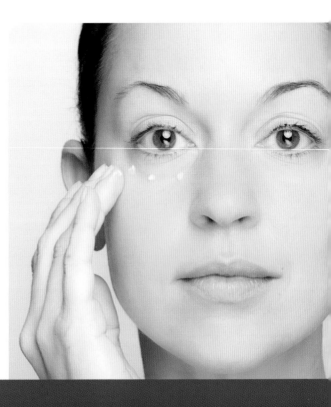

MOISTURIZERS

Once exfoliation and toning are complete, you can finally apply a moisturizer.

Moisturizers contain humectants, conditioning agents that return moisture and help to retain water in the skin. Because removing make-up can be tough on the skin, finding the right moisturizer also helps to keep the skin healthy and fresh.

The table describes the composition of moisturizers you should look for, based on your skin type.

Skin Type	Moisturizer
Dry skin	Heavier, oil-based moisturizers
Oily skin	Lighter, water-based moisturizers
Mature skin	Oil-based moisturizers
Sensitive skin	Moisturizers with soothing ingredients (such as aloe) that are fragrance and preservative free
Normal/ combination skin	Lighter, water-based moisturizers

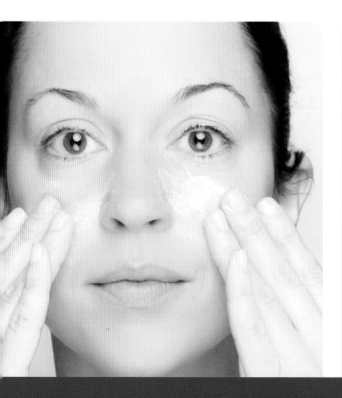

Moisturizers with SPF

Whenever possible, find a daytime moisturizer with a sun protection factor (SPF). This number refers to the theoretical amount of time you can stay in the sun without getting burned. For example, an SPF of 15 would allow you to stay in the sun 15 times longer than you could without protection. The SPF level needed depends on how fair your skin is – the fairer you are, the higher the SPF you should go with.

By using a moisturizer with SPF, you're protecting against ultraviolet (UV) radiation, the skin's worst enemy. These invisible rays are part of the energy that comes from the sun and can damage the skin, potentially leading to melanoma and other types of skin cancer.

PART 2
BREAKING DOWN YOUR LOOK

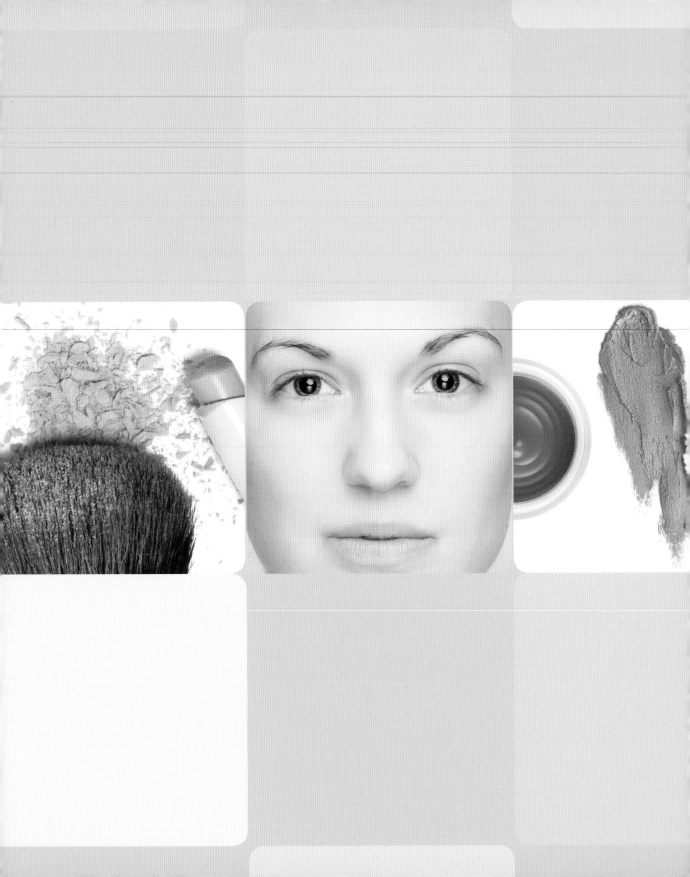

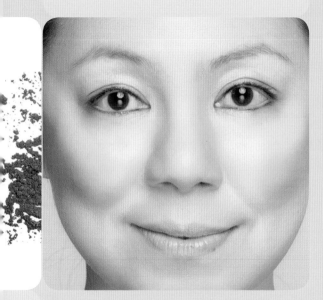

CHAPTER 4
CORRECTIVE MAKE-UP

When decorating a house, an interior designer needs to consider balance, scale, and proportion when deciding where to place furniture and accessories. These same principles apply to your make-up application. Corrective make-up is about bringing your face closer to the most attractive shape, balance, and proportion.

In this chapter, I first analyse the face and define its shape and proportions. Then I give you tips on how to highlight and contour your face to achieve the most desirable look.

ANALYSING YOUR FACE

Before you apply corrective make-up to your face, it's important to know what "corrections" you need to make.

Beyond simple spot cover-up, corrective make-up is about achieving balance and proportion and giving your face an attractive shape. So let's take a moment to break down the face and its proportions.

THE THREE FACE SEGMENTS

The face is a three-dimensional object that can be divided into equal parts. The perfect face shape has equal distances from the forehead to the eyebrow, the eyebrow to the tip of the nose, and the nose to the chin. The goal in corrective make-up is to create equality across these three segments, using highlights and shadows for balance.

FACE PROFILE

Another aspect of the three-dimensional face is the profile. There are three types of face profile: vertical, concave, and convex.

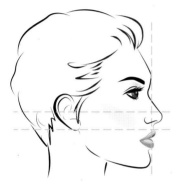 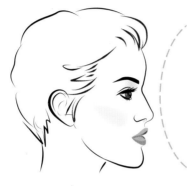 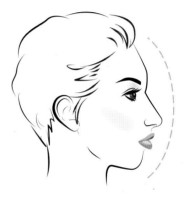

VERTICAL

This is the classic face profile. The plane between the forehead and chin runs straight up and down. This face profile does not require any corrective make-up.

CONCAVE

This profile curves inwards, with a more pronounced forehead and chin. You can create proportion within a concave profile by applying a contour colour to the forehead and chin. This will reduce those areas and balance the profile.

CONVEX

This face profile curves out like a contact lens, while the forehead and chin slope inwards and are less pronounced. By highlighting the forehead and the chin, you create the illusion of harmony and proportion. This results in a complementary relationship across the entire profile.

WIDTH OF FACE

A balanced width for the face is three eye widths across. If you remove the third eye, you have the ideal spacing between the eyes. Corrective make-up allows you to bring the eyes inwards using contour or outwards using highlighting.

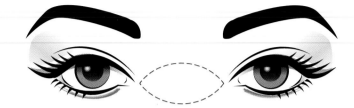

FACE SHAPE

The face shape is the surface of the front of the head from the top of the forehead to the base of the chin and from ear to ear. There are six different face shapes: oval, oblong, heart, diamond, square, and round. I'll discuss the characteristics of each face shape here; later, you'll learn how to highlight and contour according to your face shape.

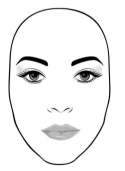

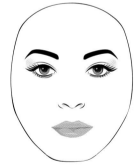

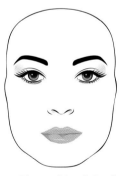

Oval: The oval face shape is a third less wide than it is long and doesn't have any major corners around the hairline or jawline. The oval face shape is round on top and curves down like an inverted egg.

Round: On a round face shape, the cheeks are the widest part of the face, with soft corners at the forehead and jawline.

Square: The width of the face at the forehead, cheekbones, and jawline are equal on a square face shape.

The "Perfect" Face

During the Renaissance, artists and architects used an equation known as the "golden ratio" to map out their masterpieces. Hundreds of years later, scientists adopted this mathematical formula to help explain why some people are considered attractive. The golden ratio is measured on a scale from 1 to 10 (with 10 considered the perfect face shape).

For the first test, divide the length of the face by the width. The ideal result is roughly 1.6, or about one and a half times longer than it is wide.

Next, the three segments of the face are measured: from the forehead hairline to a spot between the eyes, from between the eyes to the bottom of the nose, and from the bottom of the nose to the bottom of the chin. If the numbers are equal, a person is considered more attractive.

Finally, statisticians measure other facial features to determine symmetry and proportion. On an evenly balanced face, for example, the length of an ear is equal to the length of the nose, and the width of an eye is equal to the distance between the eyes.

Worried you don't have what's considered the "perfect" face? There's good news. Scientists have never found a person with a perfect score of 10!

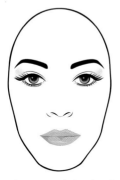

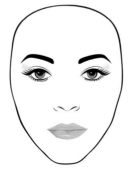

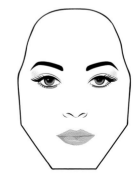

Oblong (Rectangle): This face is similar to a square; however, the oblong face shape is longer than it is wide.

Heart: This face shape is widest at the forehead and slightly less wide at the cheek, while the jawline is small and pointy.

Diamond: The diamond face shape has a narrow hairline and jawline and prominent cheekbones.

USING HIGHLIGHT AND CONTOUR

Corrective make-up is about simply using highlight (light) and contour (dark) to change the shape of the face.

Whether it's a crooked nose you would like to straighten, eyes you want to emphasize, or a strong jawline you wish to soften, corrective make-up aims to highlight features you find attractive and disguise any features you find less flattering. While full corrective make-up is quite challenging and not needed every day, some knowledge of corrective make-up will be transformative.

The rule of thumb when using corrective make-up on your face is to select a highlight one to two shades lighter and a contour one to two shades darker than your skin tone. If you'll be in a venue that's more dimly lit (such as a restaurant in the evening), you can go up to three shades lighter and darker respectively. (I will break down highlighting and contouring specific facial features in the following chapters.)

HIGHLIGHTING PRODUCTS

Highlighting is the process of lightening an area to bring it forwards or make it more prominent. The following are products you can use to achieve a highlight on the face.

Powder: You can use a light matte powder or a light shimmering powder, whether pressed or loose, to highlight features.

Cream: Cream make-up comes in tubes, pencils, and pots. It is a great choice for highlighting, because it gives a dewy glow to the skin.

CONTOURING PRODUCTS

Contour is the use of shadows or shading to reduce features on the face. It is all about the shade (the slight degree of difference between colours) you use. In most instances, you will want to choose colours that are matte, as make-up with shimmer or glitter reflects light and draws focus to the area – the opposite effect to what contour is designed to achieve.

While many cosmetic companies sell packaged "contouring" palettes, the following are some individual products you can use to contour.

Eye and cheek shadow: Matte shadows in shades of red, orange, and brown (depending on your skin tone) are popular for contouring. A pressed or loose powder shadow is a great choice for oily skin types.

Cream: Cream make-up is great for normal to dry skin types to use for contouring. Like eye shadow used for contouring, cream contour should be a shade of red, orange, or brown (depending on your skin tone).

Tinted powders: Tinted powders come in a variety of contour shades. They are sheerer than a pressed powder, which can help you achieve a more natural look.

Bronzer: If you are aiming for more of a sun-kissed look, you can use bronzer as a contour.

Corrective Make-up Note

Highlighting and contouring your face should be an illusion. Therefore, choose colours close to your skin tone to keep it looking natural. If you use a matte powder for contour and a cream for a highlighter, you will give your face a natural glow.

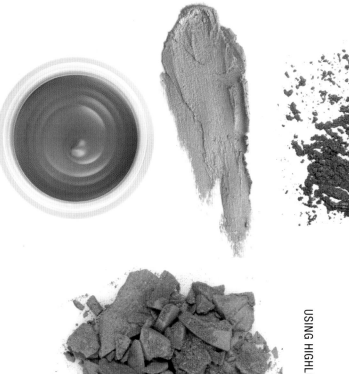

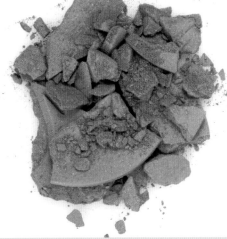

HIGHLIGHTING AND CONTOURING BY FACE SHAPE

Now that you know the parts of the face and what highlighting and contouring products you can use, it's time to learn how to highlight and contour based on your face shape. The goal of corrective make-up is to reduce orenhance portions of the face so they resemble more of an oval, which is considered the ideal face shape.

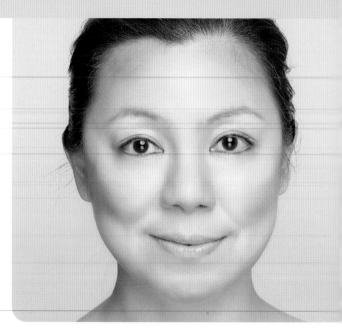

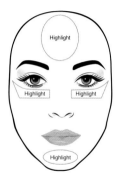

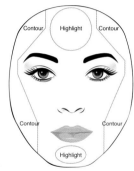

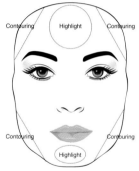

OVAL

Highlight: Apply highlight to the forehead, under the eyes, and on the chin. The highlights accentuate and brighten these areas of the oval face.

Contour: Contour is not needed, since the oval is the ideal face shape.

ROUND

Highlight: Apply highlight to the centre of the forehead and chin to draw attention to the centre of the face.

Contour: Apply contour to the jawline to reduce fullness and from the temple to the hairline to lessen the face's roundness.

SQUARE

Highlight: Apply highlight on the forehead and on the chin. This softens the strong lines of a square face.

Contour: Apply contour to both sides of the forehead and from below the ear to the jawline. This essentially reduces the "four corners" that create a square shape.

Identifying Your Face Shape

Still not sure what highlighting and contouring you need for your face? Here's quick and fun way to identify your face shape!

1. Stand in front of a mirror with overhead lighting, such as in your bathroom.

2. Pull your hair, including any fringe, back from your face.

3. Using lipstick, quickly outline your face on the mirror (excluding the ears).

4. Step back and look at the shape.

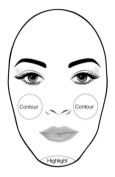

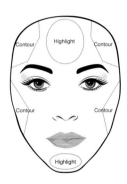

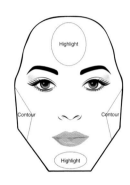

OBLONG (RECTANGLE)

Highlight: Apply highlight to the chin to draw attention to the centre of the face.

Contour: Apply contour to the cheeks to reduce the length of the face.

HEART

Highlight: Apply highlight to the centre of forehead and on either side of the chin to give the face more fullness.

Contour: Apply contour at the corners of the forehead and to the cheeks to reduce their width. It should also be applied on the bottom of the chin to soften its pointiness.

DIAMOND

Highlight: Apply highlight to the middle of the forehead and on the chin to emphasize the centre of the face. Because the diamond face shape has pronounced cheekbones, however, it does not always need a highlighter.

Contour: Apply contour to the outside of the cheekbones to diminish their width.

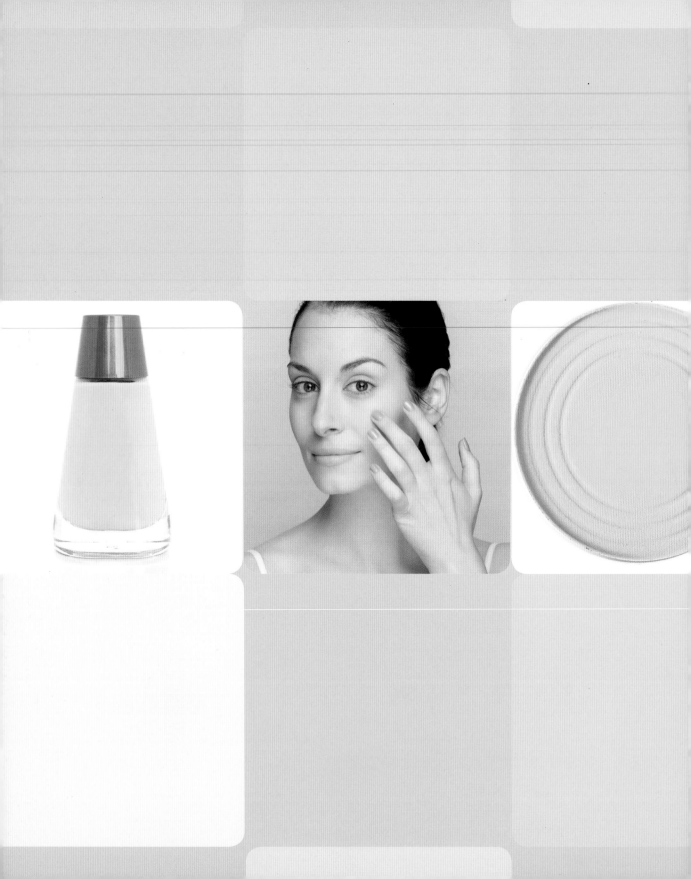

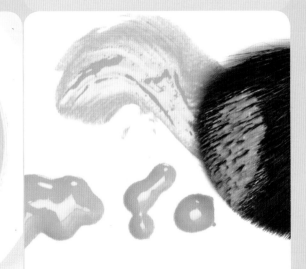

CHAPTER 5
FOUNDATION

Foundation is the first step of make-up application. It is skin-coloured make-up used to even skin tone, cover skin flaws, and sometimes even change the colour of the face. As its name denotes, it is laying the foundations for the entire application. That is why it's important to educate yourself on the correct product for you.

In this chapter, I discuss how to identify your skin tone, types of foundation and coverage, and how to apply foundation.

HOW TO IDENTIFY YOUR SKIN TONE

Human skin ranges from the darkest brown to the lightest pinkish-white.

Skin colour is a result of the body's need to protect itself from UV rays. Skin colour is affected by many substances, the primary one being melanin, which is a group of natural pigments found in most organisms. The level of skin pigmentation shows a close correspondence with latitude – people living near the equator tend to have darker skin, while lighter-skinned people mostly live nearer the poles.

Skin tone refers to the "undertone" or secondary colour of the skin. It is not what you think of as fair, olive, tan, or dark; instead, it refers to the colouring under the skin. For example, someone who has fair skin might exhibit some redness in the skin; that redness is the undertone. You may have heard skin tone referred to in terms of being a Winter, Spring, Summer, or Autumn tone. The terminology make-up artists use for skin tone is warm and cool; check out the following colour chart to see what colours comprise these skin tones.

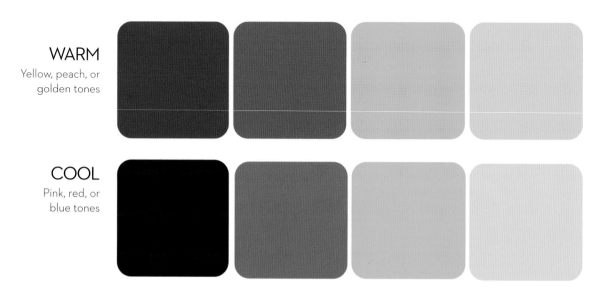

WARM
Yellow, peach, or golden tones

COOL
Pink, red, or blue tones

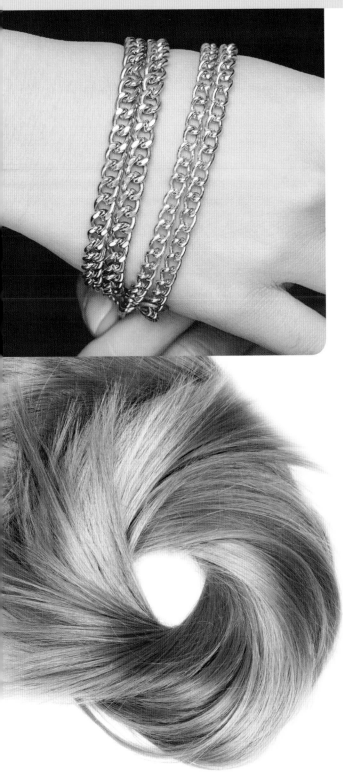

The following are some tests you can try to see if you are a warm or cool tone:

- Put on some jewellery or look at whatever jewellery you're already wearing. If you look better in gold jewellery, you most likely have warm undertones. If you look better in silver jewellery, you're more likely to have cool undertones.

- Look at the veins in your arms. If they appear greenish, you are likely to have warm undertones. If they appear blue, you have cool undertones.

- Your hair never lies! If you have copper or gold tones in your hair, you are likely to have warm undertones. If your hair is neutral to ash (blue) in colour, you are likely to have cool undertones.

- The clothes you look good in can also indicate your skin tone. If you look better in white or black fabrics, you are cool toned. If you look better in brown and off-white fabrics, you are warm toned.

- When you spend time in the sun, do you burn easily? If you do, you are most likely cool toned. However, if you tan easily, you are most likely warm toned.

Neutral Tone

Can't decide what your skin tone is, based on these tests? You may just be neutral toned. People who have neutral tones look good in all colours, though they may personally favour the colour palette of one tone over the other.

TYPES OF FOUNDATION

There are several types of foundation, and each works very differently on the skin to maximize its beauty.

The following table lists the different attributes of each of the traditional types of foundation. Take a look and see which one you think would work best for you.

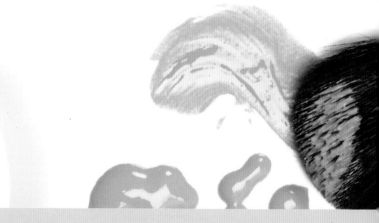

Type	Consistency	Coverage	Benefits	Finish	Skin Type	Application
Cream	Thick	Full	Covers birthmarks, pigmentation, acne, and scars	Matte	Normal, combination, dry, and mature skin	With a foundation brush, a sponge, or your fingers
Liquid	Thin	Medium	Covers flaws and provides hydration	Dewy and light	All skin types, especially dry and mature skin	With a foundation brush, a sponge, or your fingers
Pressed powder	Powder	Medium to full	Reduces shine and oil	Natural, even, and matte finishes	All skin types, especially oily	With a powder brush or sponge
Tinted	Half moisturizer and half foundation	Light to medium	Provides hydration and evens skin tone	Dewy and light	Dry and combination skin	With a foundation brush, a sponge, or your fingers

THE SPECIAL CASE OF MINERAL MAKE-UP

Beyond the options listed opposite, you can also choose to use mineral make-up. Mineral make-up comprises all the same ingredients as regular foundation (mica, titanium oxide, zinc oxide, and iron oxides). However, it contains a light sunblock and anti-inflammatory properties, and does not include parabens, preservatives, mineral oil, dyes, or fragrance, making it a healthy choice for the skin.

For skin with minimal issues, I suggest you begin by using a full-coverage foundation in place of a concealer; a full-coverage foundation will be less thick and more natural. Apply your foundation or concealer under your eyes and around the nose, and dab on any blemishes or other small areas where you want full coverage.

You can then apply your mineral foundation make-up (using a foundation brush or kabuki brush) all over your face. Blend the mineral make-up into the areas that you want concealed, and finish your look by spraying your face with a hydration mist. The end result will be beautiful, natural-looking skin.

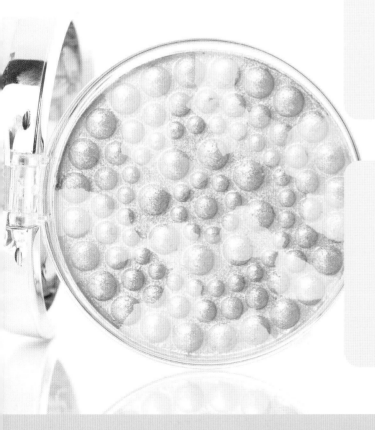

Did You Know?

While mineral make-up originally started out as a loose powder, you can now buy beautiful eye shadows, blushers, and bronzers as mineral make-up.

Using a Kabuki Brush for Mineral Make-up

A kabuki brush is a brush specifically designed for the application of mineral make-up. With its short handle and dense bristles, it is able to hold more powder for better coverage.

LEVEL OF COVERAGE

Another thing you should consider when choosing foundation is the level of coverage you'd like. There are three types of foundation coverage: sheer to light, medium, and full.

Sheer to light coverage: This type of foundation coverage is lightweight and transparent. It evens skin tone, but it won't cover flaws.

Medium coverage: With this type of coverage, you can reduce the appearance of small blemishes and uneven skin tone. However, it won't completely disguise the skin's natural colour and imperfections.

Full coverage: This type of coverage completely covers flaws and uneven skin tone. However, it can clog pores and may encourage skin breakouts.

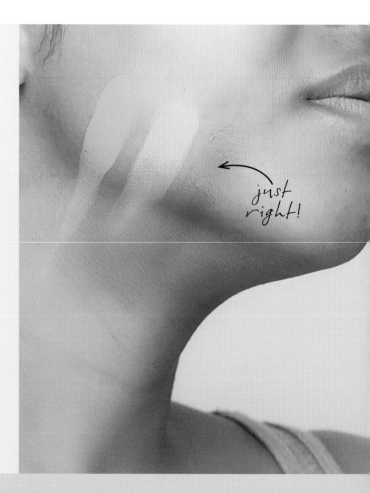

Choosing the Right Foundation

When choosing a foundation, test it on your neck leading into your jawline, rather than on your face. Your face can easily be a different shade from the rest of your body due to sun or irritation, so the goal is to match your face with your body. A good rule of thumb is to go slightly darker rather than lighter in colour if you have a fair to medium skin tone, in order to avoid looking like you have a "mask" on. On the other hand, if you have a darker skin tone, use a foundation slightly lighter than your natural skin tone to brighten your face and allow your make-up application to stand out.

just right!

FINISHES

Foundations come in three main types of finish, which can alter the look of your skin: matte, shimmer, and dewy.

Matte: Foundation with a matte finish does not contain a reflecting agent. This makes it the best product to use when contouring your face.

Shimmer: A shimmer finish foundation contains reflecting agents that draw attention to your make-up, creating a more dramatic look. Because shimmer foundation reflects light, it can be used as a highlighter above the cheekbone to the temple.

Dewy: Foundation with a dewy finish contains moisturizers to create a fresh, youthful, and luminous look. If you have mature or dry skin, it can also help your skin look more hydrated.

Making Your Own Tinted Moisturizer

To create your own tinted moisturizer, place a little concealer along with a 10p-sized amount of your favourite facial moisturizer on the back of your hand. Mix with your fingers or a cotton bud, and then apply to your face. Voilà – tinted moisturizer!

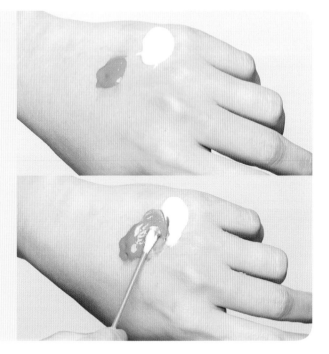

FOUNDATION TOOLS

There are three primary tools you can use to apply foundation: a sponge, a brush, or your fingers.

Whatever you decide to use, apply the foundation in downward strokes to avoid elevating fine facial hair.

SPONGES

The most common types of make-up sponge are latex and natural sponge. Latex sponges are disposable and used for a single application, while natural sponges are designed to be used multiple times. Both types of sponge can be used either dry or damp for applying foundation. Additional benefits of using a sponge include better control of the product, a sheer and lightweight application, and minimal investment.

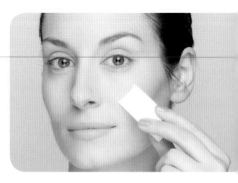

BRUSHES

I like to think of a foundation brush as a "paint brush". A foundation brush has a large head, allowing for greater coverage during application. Its bristles are synthetic, which allows for easy cleaning. The benefit of applying foundation with a brush is that it keeps the spread of bacteria (and therefore acne) to a minimum. While this brush can cause some streaking, you can stipple or tap your brush over the foundation to give a more even application.

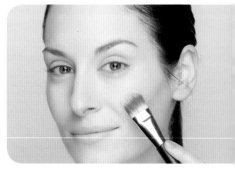

FINGERS

Fingers are the best tools you have at your disposal! Using your hands and fingers allows you to feel and control the application of foundation, resulting in better blending.

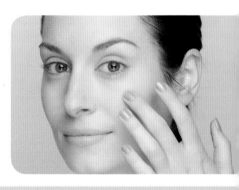

APPLYING FOUNDATION

The following walks you through how to best apply foundation.

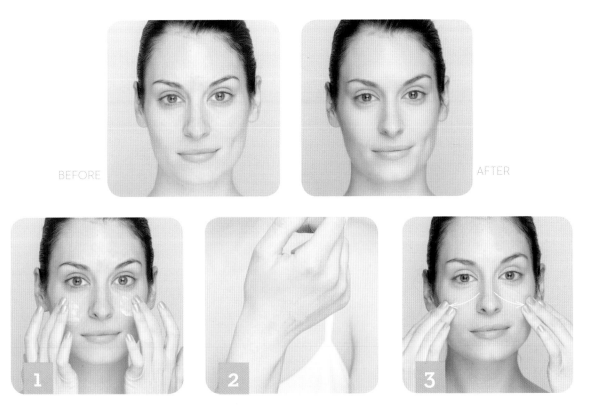

BEFORE

AFTER

1. Before you apply your foundation, moisturize your face. If you recall from my discussion of skin care, foundation will go on much more evenly when the face is moisturized.

2. Apply foundation to the back of your hand. Your hand will warm up the foundation, allowing it to go on more smoothly.

3. Swiping the foundation off your hand, start applying in the centre of your face (the sides of your nose) and work outwards. Blend the foundation evenly across your face, paying close attention to discoloured areas of skin that may need a bit more coverage.

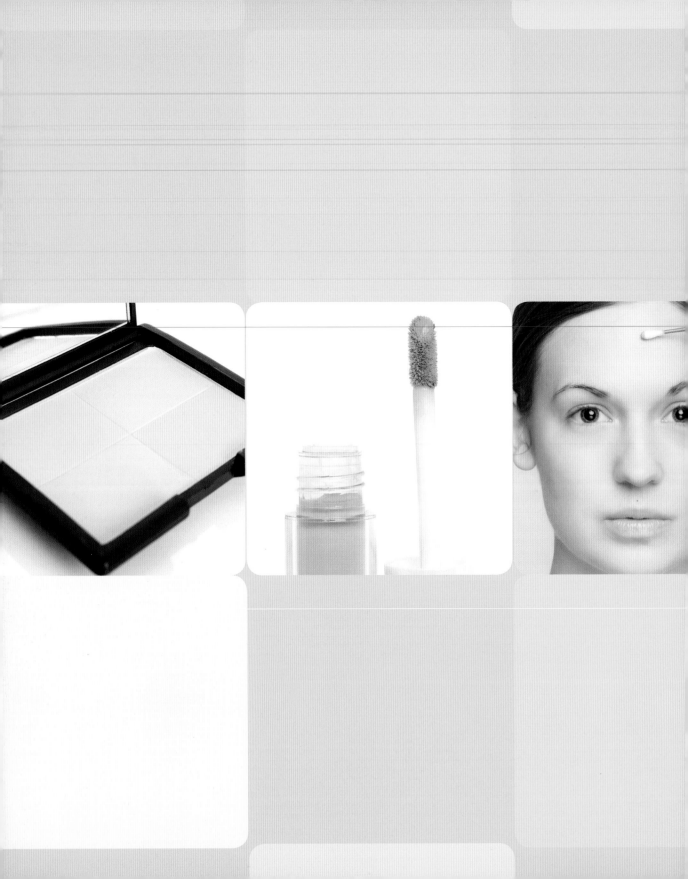

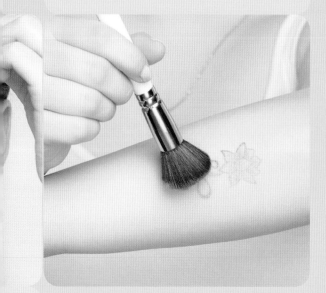

CHAPTER 6
TINTED PRIMERS, CONCEALERS, AND TATTOO COVERS

Primers, concealers, and tattoo covers are designed to provide the coverage foundation cannot. While foundations assist in evening out skin tone, they don't always provide the coverage needed to disguise blemishes or dark circles, let alone tattoos. Tinted primers are applied first to improve the coverage of your make-up and its duration. Concealers can then be used to cover dark circles, discolouration, age spots, and blemishes. And if you need to hide a tattoo, tattoo covers give you the thickness and coverage you need.

In this chapter, I discuss the products and application of tinted primers, concealers, and tattoo covers.

TINTED PRIMER

A cosmetic primer is a cream or lotion applied before concealer and foundation. Think of it as priming a wall for painting.

Using a primer can help prevent your make-up creasing and reduce the visibility of lines and crow's feet. Primer also removes colour, so the shades you want to achieve will be more successful. There are primers for the eyelids, face, and lips that are used to address discolouration from under-eye circles, blemishes, scars, and so on.

If you are experiencing discolouration and dull or lifeless skin, tinted primers can be a great choice. These come in shades that follow the law of complementary colours (other than neutral). For example, the colour red has the complementary colour of green. If you mix red and green together, you get a shade of beige/brown. Consequently, if your blemish is red and you apply a green primer, you will neutralize the colour to beige.

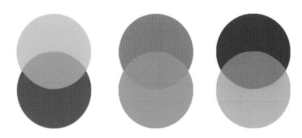

How Much?

Just a dab will do! You need only to apply the smallest amount of primer to achieve the proper results. If you apply too much, you may struggle with neutralizing the pigment.

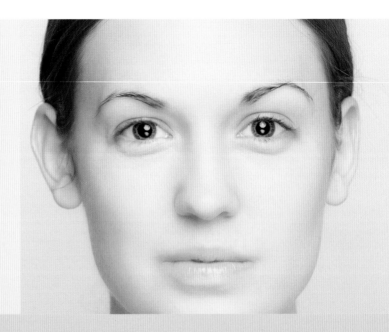

The following lists the four colours of tinted primer and how they apply the idea of complementary colours to coverage:

Red: This primer appears more pink than red, and is a great product for when your skin is sallow (yellow-green). You can also mix it with a tinted foundation to make your skin appear brighter.

Green: This primer is the complementary colour to red, meaning it's the ideal primer for neutralizing redness in the skin. You can cover a blemish or rosacea with a dab of green primer.

Yellow: This is the complementary colour to violet and is found in most highlighting creams. Yellow reflects light, giving your skin more a more glowing appearance.

Purple: The complementary colour to yellow, a thin layer of light purple primer helps reduce yellow tones in the skin. It also helps mature skin appear less dull.

CONCEALER

Concealer is a flesh-toned cosmetic product that's similar to foundation but thicker.

I consider it to be one of the most important steps in make-up application. It would be a mistake to think of concealer simply as a "cover-up". Instead, think of concealer as a play on light and a manipulation of colour. For example, if you are trying to cover dark circles (a shade or two darker than your skin colour), you need to find a concealer that is a shade or two lighter than your actual skin colour to counterbalance the discolouration.

TYPES OF CONCEALER

Concealer is full-coverage make-up that comes in liquid, cream, and powder form. Each can benefit your skin in different ways.

Liquid: This has a lighter finish and is great for dry skin. Liquid concealer can be used anywhere you need to cover imperfections. Additionally, it hydrates the under-eye area while reducing the look of dark circles and discolouration.

Cream: Much thicker than liquid concealer, a cream concealer can be used to address dark circles, spots, scars, and bruises.

Powder: Typically found in mineral make-up lines, this type of concealer is great for oily skin. Powder concealers are best used when you're dealing with a little discolouration or small skin imperfections.

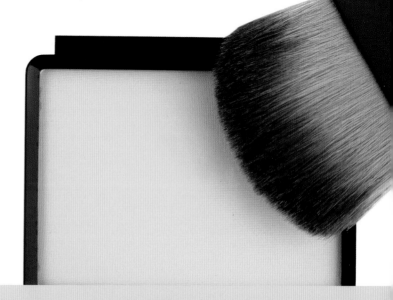

CONCEALER PACKAGING

Concealer comes in the form of sticks, compacts/containers, tubes, and pencils. The packaging is designed to assist you in easy application and spot treatment. The following is what you'll typically find with each type of concealer package.

Stick: Cream concealers typically come in a thin stick. They have a creamy consistency and are good for covering blemishes.

Compact/container: Cream and powder concealers may come in a container, either as a compact or a pot with a lid.

Tube: Liquid concealers come in a tube. You either squeeze the product out or use the applicator included in the tube (similar to a lip gloss tube).

Pencil: Pencil concealers are thicker products that come in a pencil form. They are great for spot treating areas and for concealing your lips. Be careful when applying under the eyes, however, since the skin there is thinner and requires a lighter touch.

Colour-Correcting Concealer

Colour-correcting concealer is a last resort when flesh-toned concealer doesn't work well enough to cover or neutralize severe discolourations. It is most commonly available in cream or stick form and has a thicker consistency than a tinted primer (which tends to be liquid and go on more sheer).

If you decide to try a colour-correcting concealer, apply it before foundation; this helps to neutralize and balance the unnatural colour of the product. You also can pair it with a flesh-toned concealer with the same finish, so that when the foundation is applied on top, there is no evidence of the colour corrector underneath.

The following are the different colour-correcting concealers and what they can correct, depending on your concern:

- **Lavender:** Counteracts sallowness or yellowness in the skin
- **Yellow:** Counteracts deep purple tones, such as dark circles or scarring; pale yellow also works well to highlight brows and cheekbones
- **Green:** Neutralizes redness, including redness from rosacea
- **Pink:** Neutralizes a blue cast on lighter skin tones; can also be used to enliven very pale skin
- **Orange/salmon:** Neutralizes blue to deep purple or greyish tones in deeper skin tones

APPLYING CONCEALER

Typically you apply concealer under the eyes and around the nose and mouth. Additionally, you can use concealer to cover blemishes, scars, and bruises. The following are some helpful tips on the best ways to apply concealer.

- Apply concealer under the eye with your ring finger, which tends to have the lightest touch. You can place it right below the tear ducts by tapping it lightly in a U-shaped pattern from the inside to the outside of the eye.

- Use an angle or eyeliner brush to dab concealer on the top of any blemishes. Doing so helps to concentrate the product on top of the blemish.

- To reduce the look of puffy eyes, use a hydrating (liquid) concealer two shades lighter than your skin tone and apply it under the eye with your ring finger, a brush, or a beauty sponge.

Other Concealer Tips and Tricks

Concealer can be your best friend. Here are some concealer tips to help your make-up appear flawless!

- **Are you having a difficult time covering your dark under-eye circles?** Use a hydrating eye cream to plump up the under-eye area before applying your concealer.

- **Want to get rid of those fine lines?** All you need is a wrinkle-filling serum and some liquid concealer. Squeeze a bit of the wrinkle filler onto your finger, dab it into the wrinkle, and blend until it is barely noticeable. You can then top with the liquid concealer to completely hide that fine line.

- **Experiencing problems with covering uneven skin tone?** You don't want to overdo the concealing when you have uneven skin tone, as this can look extremely unflattering and unnatural. So start with a full-coverage foundation and apply it with a clean foundation brush or sponge. From there, dot on your yellow-based concealer and blend.

- **Would you like to wear that fabulous skirt, but you're afraid to expose those pesky spider veins on your body?** Use a pencil or wand-style concealer (in your skin tone), which will allow for the most coverage and control, and trace over the veins. Blend the concealer with your little finger and set with some pressed translucent powder.

- **Do you have a red and irritated nose due to a cold or allergies?** To get rid of the redness first, avoid moisturizer; instead, just use a flat-tipped concealer brush or cotton bud to apply a bit of yellow-based concealer right around the red areas of your nose. Next, really blend on your foundation to neutralize the rest of the redness. Finally, cover it up with a bit of translucent powder.

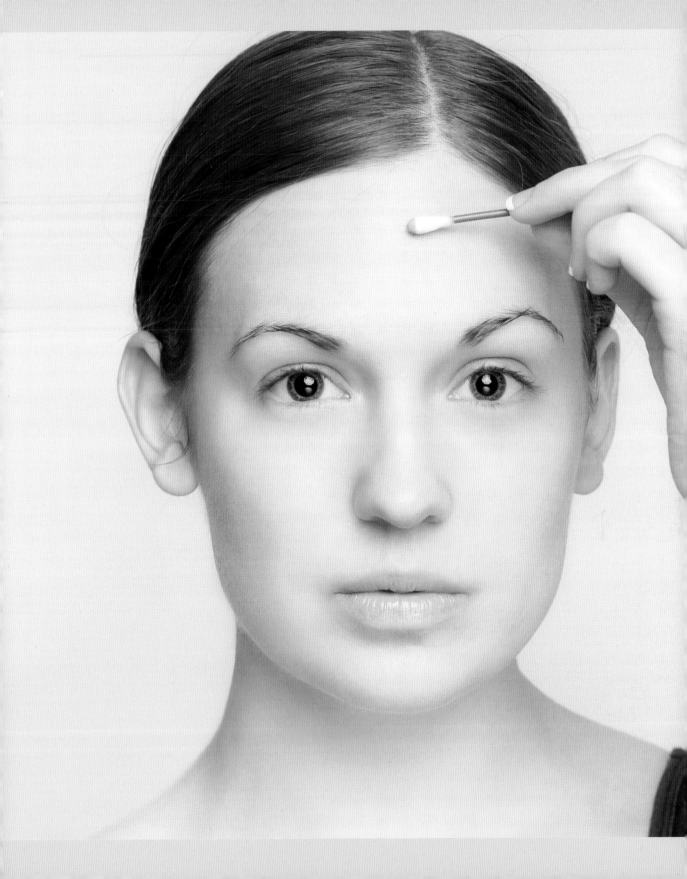

TATTOO COVER

Have you ever tried to cover a tattoo for a wedding or a formal function?

Foundations and concealers don't work well because they are usually sheer, slightly translucent, and simply won't cover the ink.

When you need to cover a tattoo, the product you want to use is tattoo cover (sometimes called *camouflage cover*). Tattoo cover has the same effect as a concealer, with the main difference being simply thickness. Tattoo cover is very thick and opaque with a matte finish to cover up the dark and multicoloured inks used in tattoos. Stores sell tattoo wheels or palettes with multiple shades. Because skin isn't typically one colour, multiple shades are helpful in creating a more realistic look.

Ready to try covering your tattoo? The following walks you through how to do so.

Can't Find Tattoo Cover?

If you do not have access to tattoo cover, you can use a full-coverage foundation or even theatrical make-up. However, you may need a few extra layers to achieve the desired coverage.

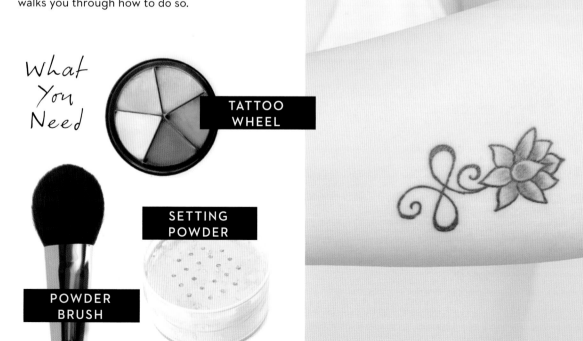

What You Need

TATTOO WHEEL

SETTING POWDER

POWDER BRUSH

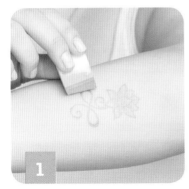

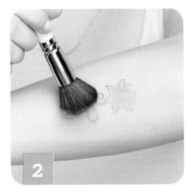

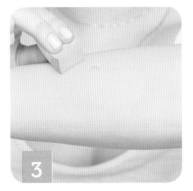

1 Choose a shade lighter than your skin colour and press the cover-up into the area. You do not want to rub or brush the product onto your skin, as it will move around, making it difficult to fully cover the tattoo.

2 Use a setting powder to set the tattoo cover. If you can still see the tattoo, repeat the steps, covering the tattoo with the same shade of tattoo cover and then setting again with powder.

3 Choose three different shades of tattoo cover – one closest to your skin colour, one slightly lighter, and one slightly darker. Using your fingers or a porous sponge, tap the shades over the area of your tattoo. This will replicate the different tones in the skin. Powder the area and repeat the process of tapping in the colour shades as many times as necessary. Once you are left with a circle of product on your tattoo, blend the edges of the tattoo cover into your skin to even it out.

Gone!

Liquid Skin

Liquid Skin is designed as a liquid bandage, but it also works as a good base for tattoo cover application. Apply a thin layer of it over your tattoo and allow it to dry before following the steps for covering your tattoo. Liquid Skin is available from the first-aid section of most pharmacies.

TATTOO COVER

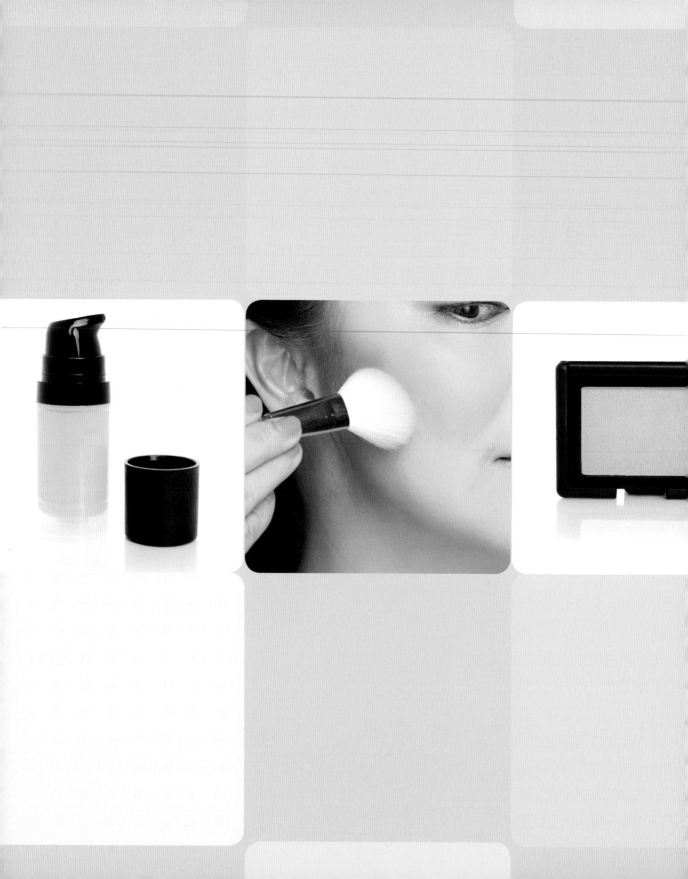

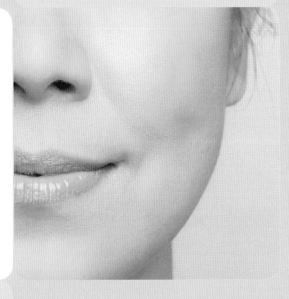

CHAPTER 7
CHEEKS

The cheeks are an important aspect of any make-up look. Cheek colour can add a glow, change the face shape, and create drama. Everyone has the right to have amazing cheekbones! Do you feel your cheekbones are nonexistent? Are you uncertain about which cheek colour is right for you?

In this chapter, I discuss different cheek colour products, as well as how to create beautiful cheekbones, based on your face shape and through the application of highlight, contour, and cheek colour.

CHEEK COLOUR PRODUCTS

Cheek colour comes in several different shades, typically belonging to the red and orange families.

This pop of colour can provide a healthy glow and give your face more balance. You can find cheek colour in cream, powder, or mineral forms. Take a look at each type and see which is right for you.

Choosing the Right Colour for Your Cheeks

Cheek colour comes in warm and cool shades, so when choosing a colour, consider your undertone, as discussed in Chapter 5. The wrong colour could make or break your final look. A good rule of thumb is to match your cheek colour to your lip colour.

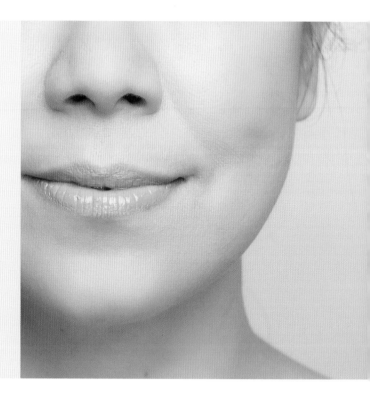

Cream: This type of cheek colour goes on sheer and provides a dewy look to the cheek. It should be applied with a synthetic blusher brush, a sponge, or your fingers. Use cream colour if you have normal or dry skin.

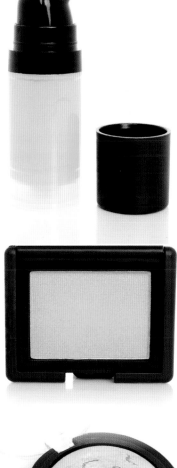

Powder: This cheek colour tends to be more matte in finish and is applied to the cheeks with a blusher brush. Powder cheek colour is great for oily skin.

Mineral: This cheek colour, applied with a blusher or kabuki brush, is easy to blend with mineral foundation. It goes on sheer and illuminates the cheeks. Mineral cheek colour is good for all skin types, especially sensitive and mature skin.

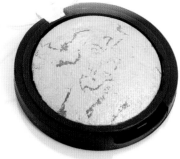

Bronzer: This type of cheek colour provides a natural, sun-kissed glow without exposing your skin to harmful UV rays. Like other cheek colours, bronzer comes in cream, powder, and mineral forms. Matte bronzers also make an excellent contour. Depending on its consistency, you can apply bronzer with a blusher brush, a sponge, or your fingers.

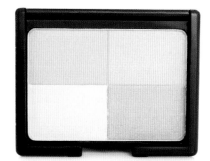

HIGHLIGHTING AND CONTOURING YOUR CHEEKS

If you choose to contour anything on your face, I would consider the cheeks to be at the top of the list.

A great cheek/cheekbone changes your face shape and directs the emphasis to the middle of your face. Plus, if you think your face is too round or your cheeks are too plump, you can rectify any problems and get the "supermodel cheeks" you crave. To change the shape of a cheekbone, just as you've learned about corrective make-up in general, you need a lighter shade (highlight) and a darker shade (contour).

Highlight: Highlighting brings emphasis to an area. Your highlight colour should be a half to full shade lighter than your skin tone. Highlight colours come in powder and cream.

- *Powder highlight* is a great choice for those with oily skin. Some products include a shimmer for additional glow.

- *Cream highlight* provides more hydration for those with normal to dry skin. Cream highlights naturally look shinier than powder, which makes them a great choice.

Contour: Because contouring creates a shadow effect, your contour colour should be a half to full shade darker than your natural skin tone. You can use either matte powder or matte cream.

- *Powder contour* is a great choice for those with oily skin and goes on naturally matte.

- *Cream contour* provides more hydration for those with normal to dry skin. Cream is also easy to blend.

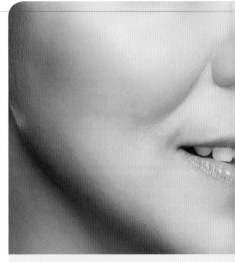

Cheeks in High Definition

Mix a cream cheek colour with a little of your foundation and then apply it to your cheeks. The cream colour will blend better with the foundation, giving your face a more uniform look.

If you choose to change the shape of your cheeks, you can follow these three easy steps.

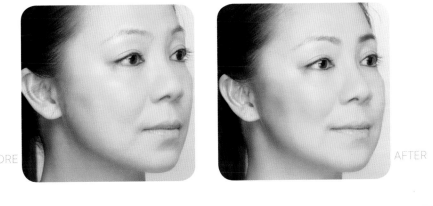

BEFORE AFTER

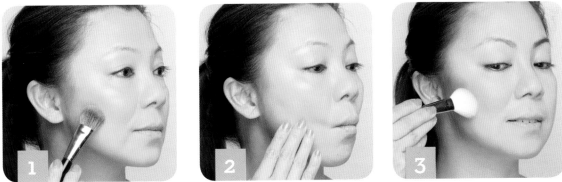

1. Look into the mirror while you suck in your cheeks. With a blusher brush, apply your contour from the bottom of the cheekbone to above the jawline. This helps to reduce the area of the cheek you want to appear slimmer.

2. Use your fingers to feel where your cheekbone starts under the centre of your eye, moving back to your temple. Add a light powder or cream as a highlight to make this area more prominent. This also brightens the eye area while providing definition.

3. Apply your cheek colour to the area between the highlight and the contour, and then blend all three together.

APPLYING HIGHLIGHT, CONTOUR, AND BLUSHER BY FACE SHAPE

Now that you know about highlighting and contouring your cheeks, as well as how to change the shape of your cheeks, it's time to bring these together.

The following shows you how to apply highlight, contour, and blusher, based on your face shape.

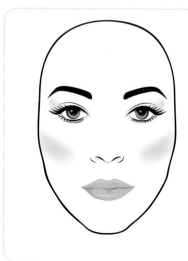

OVAL

Remember, oval is the ideal face shape. Therefore, highlight and contour will not be needed unless you want to accentuate the hollows of the cheeks or upper cheekbones. The ideal placement of cheek colour would be to apply the blusher across the cheekbones; however, keep it to just under the outside of the eye, not to the temples. Because your facial features are balanced, there's no need to apply blusher lower on your face – this would make the jaw look heavier.

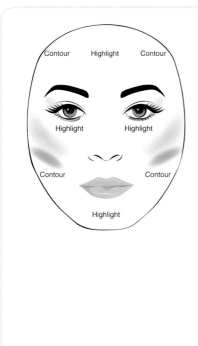

ROUND

The goal for a round face is to reduce the roundness of the cheeks by cutting the cheeks in half – colourwise, of course.

Highlight: Apply highlight to the centre of the face – the forehead, under the eyes, and the chin – to draw attention to these areas. Avoid highlight on the cheekbones, especially in the temple area; highlights here will only make the area more pronounced.

Contour: Apply contour in the hollows of the cheeks. Add contour in a diagonal line to visually divide the cheeks in half, thus reducing the roundness of the cheeks.

Blusher: Apply the desired cheek colour in between the highlight and contour.

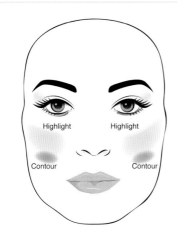

SQUARE

For the square face shape, you're basically doing the opposite of the round face shape – creating roundness instead of diminishing it. This softens an otherwise strong face shape.

Highlight: Apply highlight above the cheekbones on a diagonal to soften the strong lines of the face.

Contour: Apply contour to the hollows of the cheeks, creating a thin oval on the diagonal line. The slight oval creates roundness in the lower cheeks.

Blusher: Apply blusher in a circular motion from the temple down to the apples of the cheeks, almost like drawing a tick mark on the cheeks. This helps to create further roundness in the cheeks.

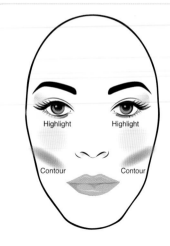

OBLONG (RECTANGLE)

The longest of the face shapes is the oblong face shape. The goal with this shape is to shorten the face while also creating softness in the cheek area, as with the square face shape.

Highlight: Apply highlight from the temple to under the eyes, using a diagonal line to soften the face shape.

Contour: Apply contour to the diagonal line in the hollow part of the cheeks. This gives the illusion of roundness.

Blusher: Apply colour in a circular manner close to the apples of the cheeks to continue softening the facial features.

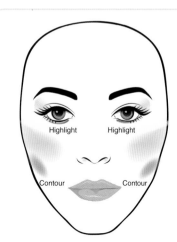

HEART

The heart face shape is wider at the top and narrower at the bottom. Your goal is to reduce some of the width at the top of the face to balance the narrow chin.

Highlight: Apply a slight horizontal highlight above the cheekbones to focus attention on this area.

Contour: Apply contour just under the cheeks and blend downwards to add a bit of fullness to the jawline.

Blusher: Apply colour between the highlight and contour on a slight horizontal. This gives the illusion of less space between the eyes.

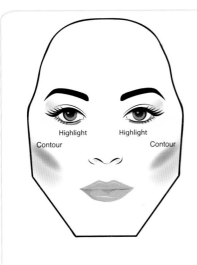

DIAMOND

The strongest feature of the diamond face shape is the cheekbones. Therefore, the goal is to make your prominent cheeks appear to be moving back into the face.

Highlight: Because the cheekbones are already prominent, keep your highlight under the eyes, sweeping it slightly up and out.

Contour: Apply contour, such as a bronzer, into the cheekbones to recede the cheeks into the face shape.

Blusher: Apply blusher just below the contour to finish off your look.

More Tips for Applying Blusher!

- Most brushes that come with a blusher are useless. Throw them out and invest in a blusher brush that is slightly larger than the apples of your cheeks.
- Cream blusher can be used on the lips for a complementary sheer and soft look.
- Powder blusher should always be applied in one direction to avoid streaking.
- To find out the actual position of the apple of your cheek, look into the mirror, smile, and then sweep a blusher brush upwards in an arc from your cheekbone to your hairline.
- Some dark blusher on the tip of your nose will make it look shorter. Blend the colour in gently.
- For a natural look, use cream blusher with cream foundation, or powder blusher with a powder foundation.

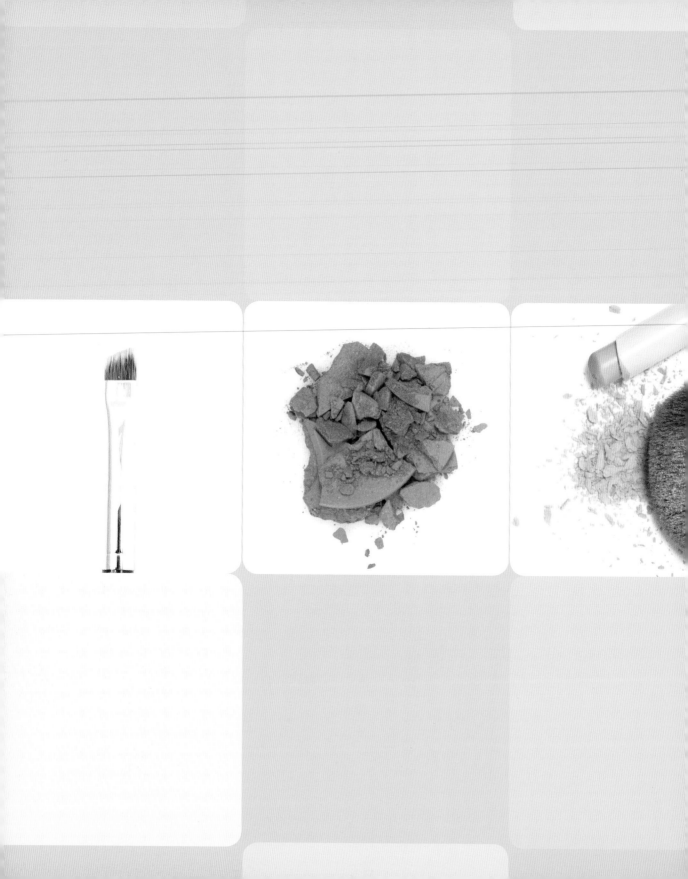

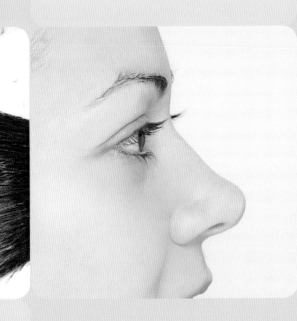

CHAPTER 8
NOSE

The nose is very important to facial symmetry because it's the centre of the face. In art design, we use the term *emphasis*, which refers to where we want to draw a viewer's attention. You don't have to spend thousands of pounds on plastic surgery if you think your nose is too distracting, whatever its shape or size. Using the magic of highlight and contour, you can give your nose the perfect proportions!

In this chapter, I address the different nose shapes and the corrective techniques you can use to make your nose complement your face.

WHAT YOU SHOULD KNOW ABOUT YOUR NOSE

The nose is divided into four main areas: the bridge, sidewalls, tip, and nostrils.

When it comes to creating the most balanced look, your nose should be in proportion to the rest of your face. What does that involve? The following are guidelines to the ideal length and width of your nose.

Length of the nose: From the centre of the eyebrows to the tip of the nose should be equal to the distance from the hairline to the brow and the tip of the nose to the chin.

Width of the nose: The edge of the nostrils should be directly below the tear ducts of the eyes.

NOSE HIGHLIGHT AND CONTOUR SHADES AND TOOLS

You can correct a wide, thin, or even a crooked nose with highlight and contour.

Let's first go over what you need to accomplish this.

Contour: Use a powder or cream colour that's a half to full shade darker than your natural skin or foundation colour.

Highlight: Use a powder or cream colour that's a half to full shade lighter than your natural skin or foundation colour.

Angle brush or small shadow brush: An angle brush will give a more precise line down the bridge of your nose, while a small shadow brush will create a softer line down it. Additionally, you can use the small shadow brush to blend the contour.

Disposable make-up sponge or beauty sponge: You can use a damp disposable make-up sponge or the smallest point of a damp beauty sponge to blend nose highlight and contour.

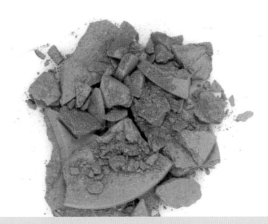

HIGHLIGHTING AND CONTOURING YOUR NOSE BY NOSE SHAPE

Whether your nose is too long for your face or you want to "fix" a crooked nose, I can help!

Highlighting and contouring using an angle brush, a small eye shadow brush, and/or a sponge can address various nose shapes and concerns. Remember, these corrections should be subtle, especially for daytime make-up. The following shows you how to slim down a wide nose, widen a thin nose, shorten a long nose, lengthen a short nose, and straighten a crooked nose. Natural noses don't need any highlighting or contouring.

WIDE

If you have a wide nose, the goal is to reduce the appearance of the width of the nose. This can be achieved by reducing the sidewalls and emphasizing the centre of the nose.

Highlight: Apply highlight straight down the bridge at the width and length you would like your nose to be. This placement helps the nose appear thinner.

Contour: Apply a shadow or darker foundation to the sides of the nose, using the side of your tool to create a line down each side of the highlight. Blend the contour down the sidewalls to complete the look.

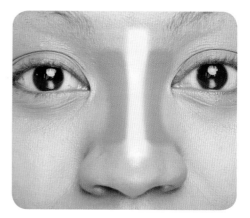

Highlighting Caution

Be careful not to make the highlight line on your nose's bridge too thin. You don't want your nose to look like a toothpick!

THIN

If you have a thin nose, you can use make-up to create the appearance of more width. Widening the highlight past the sidewalls achieves this look.

Highlight: Apply highlight just past the bridge of the nose.

Contour: Apply shadow, darker foundation, or bronzer to the nose, using the side of the brush to create a line down each side of the highlight. These lines should run past the bridge into the sidewalls. Drag the contour brush down the sidewalls to finish.

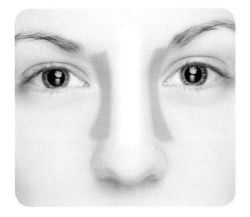

LONG

With long noses, reducing the appearance of length is the primary goal. This is achieved by stopping the highlight at the desired length of the nose.

Highlight: Starting at the top of the bridge, apply highlight down the bridge of the nose. Do not extend the highlight onto the tip of the nose; stopping short of the tip prevents the eye travelling downwards.

Contour: Apply contour just under the tip of the nose, being careful not to blend it too far onto the tip. Too much contour can make your nose look dirty.

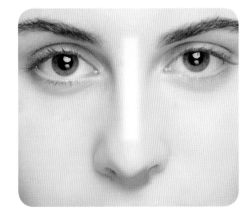

SHORT

For a short nose, the goal is to lengthen its appearance. In this case, highlight is pulled to the tip of the nose and contour extends onto the nostrils.

Highlight: Starting at the top of the bridge, drag highlight down to the tip of the nose to visually create length.

Contour: Apply contour to the sides of the nose. Bring the contour all the way down the nose to the nose's tip (following the highlight) to finish.

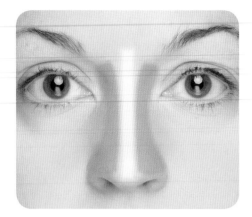

CROOKED

Even if your nose is crooked, highlight and contour can "fix" it, giving the appearance of a straight nose.

Highlight: Imagine where the line of a straight nose should be. Drag highlight straight down to the tip of the nose following this imaginary line. It's okay if you overlap the sidewalls; highlight corrects the shadows that define a crooked nose.

Contour: Using your applied highlight line as a guide, apply contour on either side of this new line. Blend contour down the sidewalls to finish.

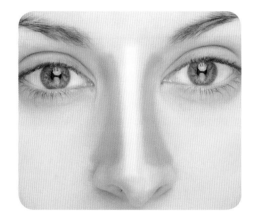

NOSE

Tips for Different Nose Concerns

- **Flat nose:** Apply highlight down the centre of the nose, avoiding the sides. Smooth and blend down the centre.

- **Broad nose:** To slim this down, sweep a foundation one shade darker than your natural skin tone along the sides of the nose with a small, firm make-up brush. Start just below the inner corners of the eyebrows and end at the sides of the nostrils. Stroke a lighter shade of foundation down the bridge of the nose. Blend well.

- **Narrow nose:** Sweep concealer that's slightly darker than your natural skin tone down the centre of the nose. Apply a lighter shade on the sides of the nose and nostrils.

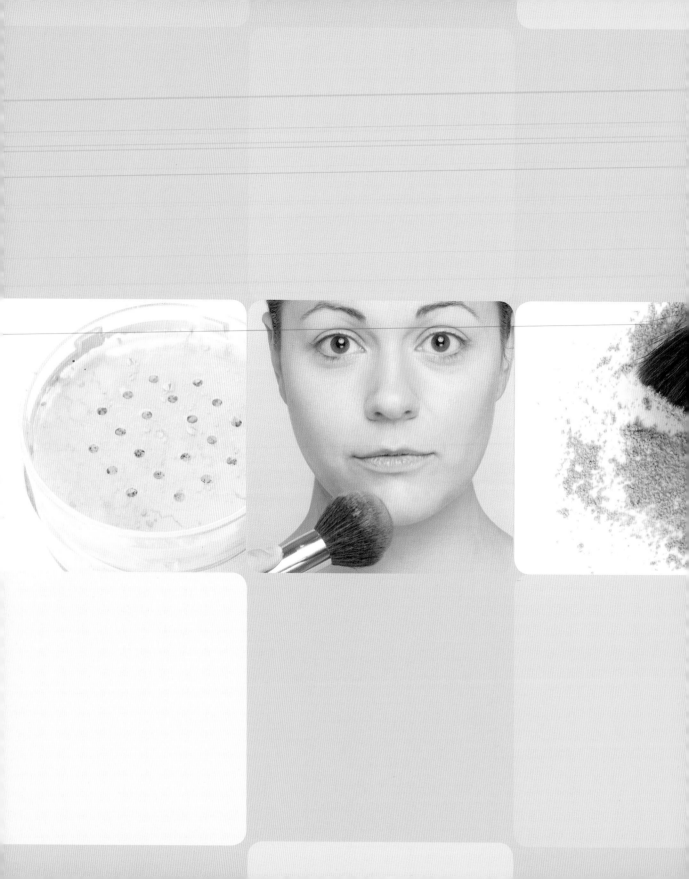

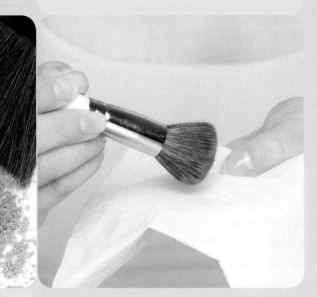

CHAPTER 9
SETTING
POWDER

After applying concealer and foundation and contouring your face, cheeks, and nose, it's time to apply setting powder. Setting powder is used to reduce oil and sweat on your face, set cream foundation, and blend your highlight and contour – in other words, it "sets" your face make-up.

In this chapter, I take you through the types of setting powder available, what you can use to put it on, and the best way to apply it.

TYPES OF SETTING POWDER

There are several types of setting powder that work well on their own for normal to oily skin types. Mineral powder works well for all skin types.

The following are the basic types available, along with the advantages of each type.

Pressed powder: This comes in a compact and is great for absorbing oil on the skin, reducing shine, and setting your foundation.

Loose powder: This is similar to pressed powder, but it's more finely milled. This means you can layer a loose powder for better coverage. Loose powder typically comes in a shaker container; holes in the container's top help to control the amount of product you are using and contain spillage.

Translucent powder: This is a setting powder that does not contain pigment, so you can set your foundation without competing with the foundation's base colour. Translucent powder works on any skin colour.

Tinted setting powder: This is tinted in shades that complement various skin colours, adding a little colour when you are not using a foundation. In addition, it is great for helping blend corrective make-up. I personally use tinted setting powder on my clients to blend out the highlights and contouring I create in a make-up application.

Mineral powder: This powder absorbs excess oil and reduces shine. Because mineral make-up is tinted and creates a glowing look, I often use it as a setting powder. The trick is to use a foundation brush versus a kabuki brush. Foundation brushes have fewer bristles, which leave less powder on the skin than a kabuki brush.

Avoiding Pressed Powder Breakage

Having trouble with your pressed powder staying together? Place a cotton wool ball or pad in your powder compact to keep your pressed powder from breaking in your make-up bag.

POWDER APPLICATION TOOLS

Setting powder can be applied with a powder puff, a powder brush, or even a kabuki brush. It all depends on how heavily you want the powder to go on and how you prefer to blend it.

Powder puff: A powder puff typically comes with any pressed or loose powder. It's made of a soft material that's used to press powder into the skin. You can also use the powder puff to blend contours and highlights into the skin after you apply your setting powder. Because reusing a powder puff will cause oil and debris to transfer from the face to the compact, consider investing in a powder puff that you can hand or machine wash.

Powder brush: The largest of the brushes, a powder brush has longer hairs to dust the setting powder onto your skin. It is easier to clean than a powder puff and can be used with all setting powder products. However, it is especially effective with loose powder because the longer and less dense brush provides a lighter application.

Kabuki brush: Because of its short, dense hairs, you have the option of using this brush to blend your make-up with the setting powder.

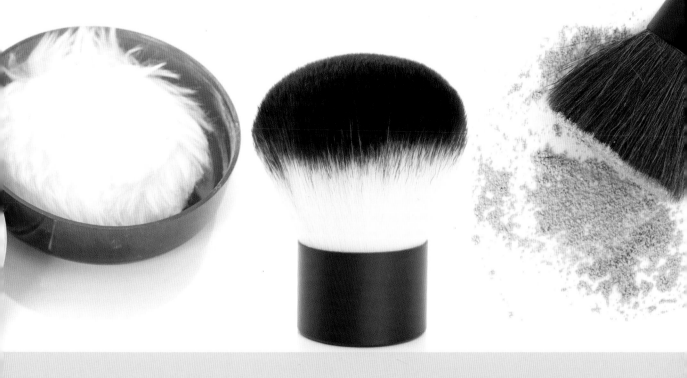

APPLYING SETTING POWDER

Setting powder has several functions, such as setting make-up so it doesn't come off, and blending your highlight and contour into your skin.

It is not about providing more coverage, like a foundation or concealer; the setting powder should simply give your face a softer look and help the foundation and concealer to stay on longer.

BASIC APPLICATION

The following is a basic application of setting powder, which mirrors foundation application. Use a light hand so as not to remove the foundation and concealer beneath.

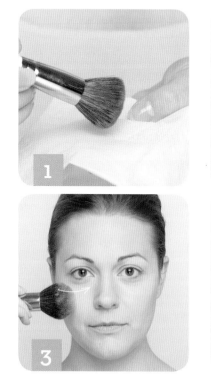

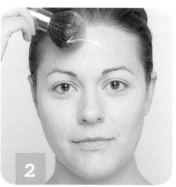

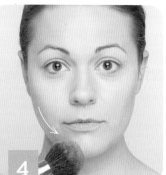

1. Tap any excess powder off the powder brush.

2. Apply the setting powder starting at the forehead and brushing back and forth horizontally.

3. Move your brush down the side of the nose and horizontally under the eye.

4. Move your brush horizontally over the cheek and down to the chin. Repeat on the opposite side.

BLENDING HIGHLIGHTS AND CONTOURS

You have the option of using tinted or translucent setting powder to blend your highlight and contour, so they don't sit on top of your foundation and concealer. Unlike the basic application, you are pressing rather than brushing the powder into the skin to effectively blend in the highlight and contour.

BEFORE

AFTER

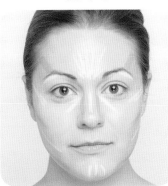

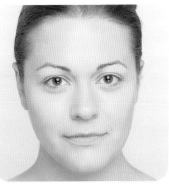

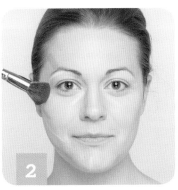

Using a Hydrating Mist

If you want your make-up to last longer, spray your face with a hydrating mist after applying your setting powder. The water more fully sets the powder into your skin.

1. Press your powder puff or kabuki brush into the setting powder.

2. Press the powder into the skin; do not brush back and forth. You are essentially pushing the highlight and contour colour into the foundation, otherwise known as blending your make-up.

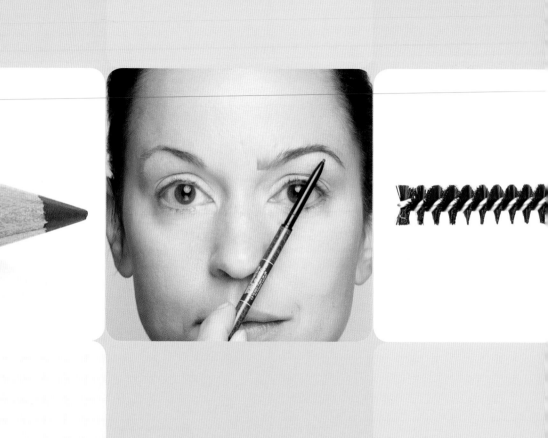

CHAPTER 10
EYEBROWS

If the eyes are the windows to the soul, then eyebrows are the frames to those windows! You can create a beautiful eye shadow application, but the look will fall short if your eyebrows are not shaped and shaded correctly. This makes it critical to have your eyebrows looking their best.

This chapter focuses on the types of eyebrow for your face shape, brow shaping techniques, and how to fill in your brows.

THE PERFECT EYEBROW

Before I get into grooming and shaping your eyebrows, let's talk about where your eyebrow should start, angle, and end.

Using a make-up brush, we're going to identify the three points of the perfect eyebrow.

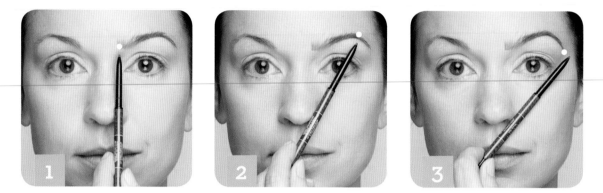

1. Hold your make-up brush vertically along the side of your nose. This is where your eyebrow should begin.

2. Pivot your brush off your nose until it crosses your pupil. This will be the highest point of your arch. Your brow should arch on an angle to the right or left of your pupil – not above it!

3. Hold your make-up brush at an angle from your nose to the outside corner of your eye. This is where your brow should end.

Shaping Overtweezed Brows

Have you overtweezed your eyebrows to the point where you can no longer see their shape? I suggest drawing your "future" eyebrow over your current brow using an eye pencil or an eye shadow with an angle brush. You can even take a picture if you need to remember the shape. Once that's done, tweeze around the drawn eyebrow. It may take weeks to see the desired brow shape, but it's worth the wait!

EYEBROW TYPES

You may not realize it, but the shape of your eyebrows can be a key element in a successful make-up look.

There are five different eyebrow shapes you can have or sculpt – round, angled, soft angled, curved, and flat.

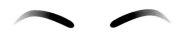

ROUND

A round eyebrow is an even curve without points.

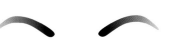

ANGLED

An angled eyebrow comes to more of a peak before sloping downwards. It's a stronger eyebrow than the traditional round shape.

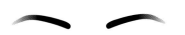

SOFT ANGLED

A soft-angled eyebrow is similar to an angled one. However, instead of coming to a strong point, it curves slightly at its peak.

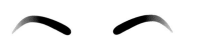

CURVED

A curved eyebrow has two curves – a smaller upside-down U, followed by a larger curve over the brow bone.

FLAT

A flat eyebrow does not have a strong peak. The brow is more horizontal, with a subtle slope at the end.

THE BEST EYEBROWS FOR EACH FACE SHAPE

My favourite moment as a make-up artist is when I reshape my clients' brows.

It frames their eye make-up, balances their face shape, and adds that perfect pop of drama. I'd like to show you how to perfect your face shape with a suitable eyebrow shape.

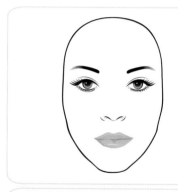

OVAL

While any eyebrow shape can work, soft-angled brows are the most attractive on this versatile face shape. Soft-angled brows complement the natural curve of an oval face.

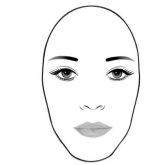

OBLONG (RECTANGLE)

Flat brows work best on the oblong face shape. This is because a long face needs more balance than any other shape, which thick, straight brows can provide. These brows are also helpful in not accentuating the length of the face, unlike arched brows.

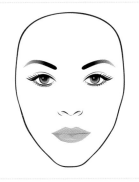

HEART

People with heart-shaped faces should ideally have rounded or curved brows. These brows help balance the pointy chin. Stay away from flat brows, which tend to overaccentuate the chin instead.

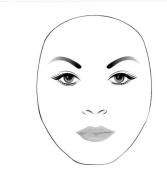

SQUARE

Curved or angled brows are recommended for a square-shaped face, which needs softening for the four corners. Both brow types soften and balance the symmetry of this face shape. Avoid an overly arched brow shape, as it can create an exaggerated jawline.

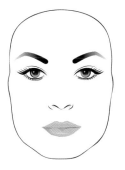

ROUND

Round faces look good with angled or soft-angled brows. Either brow can add length and strength to the face shape. Having the arch of the brows taper to a sharp point makes the cheekbones appear higher and the jawline look more distinct, for an overall elongating effect.

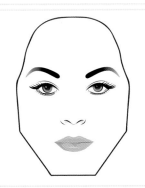

DIAMOND

A diamond face shape requires brows that balance the strong cheekbones. With this face shape, you should go with round, curved, or angled brows to narrow the face.

THE BEST EYEBROWS FOR EACH FACE SHAPE

BROW SHAPING

The perfect brow shape does wonders for your face.

Now that you know which brow works best with your features, it's time to look at how to shape your brows. While you're free to seek the help of a professional for this, there are a couple of quick and easy ways you can shape your brows from the comfort of your own home: tweezing and waxing.

Tweezing: Using tweezers, a slender metal tool with a pointed or flat end, you pluck one hair at a time until you create the shape you desire. Be careful not to overpluck your eyebrows, or you'll end up having to shade them in.

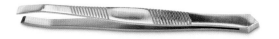

Waxing: This requires a pot of heated wax and a wooden spatula. The spatula is dipped into heated wax, and then the wax is applied to the area on the brow where you'd like to remove hair. After a few moments, you pull it off in the opposite direction to the hair growth. There are two kinds of wax used with this technique: soft and hard wax.

Soft wax is the consistency of honey. When heated, it can be applied with a wooden spatula and removed with a cloth strip. It removes the hair quickly. While redness often follows a soft wax, it should go away within an hour. You can apply aloe afterwards to reduce redness and irritation.

Hard wax is a great option for those with sensitive skin or on acne medication, which can make the skin thin and easily irritated. This technique does not require a cloth for removal. The wax dries, holding the hair in the product. You then simply pull the hard wax off, removing the hairs with it.

Threading

Originating in India, threading is a fast and inexpensive brow-shaping technique that has become very popular internationally. In threading, a thin cotton thread is doubled, twisted, and then rolled across areas where the hair needs to be removed. This motion pulls the hair out at the follicle, one hair at a time.

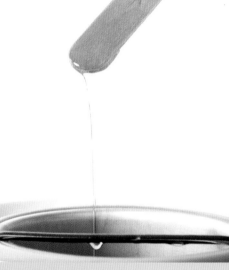

Waxing at Home

Not getting the eyebrow waxing results you want? Follow these steps, using the products indicated (which you can find at beauty supply shops or online), and you'll end up with perfectly waxed eyebrows every time!

Small cosmetic scissors

Prewax cleanser

Baby powder

Wax applicator (such as a wooden spatula)

Heated soft wax

Muslin cloth strips

Baby oil or wax remover

Aloe vera

1. Before waxing, pull your hair back from your face and decide which eyebrow shape will suit your features best. If necessary, trim your eyebrows with small cosmetic scissors.

2. Apply prewax cleanser to your eyebrows; this will help avoid any infection.

3. Dab baby powder on your eyebrows. This acts as a barrier between the wax and your skin.

4. Using your eyebrow wax applicator, apply wax in the direction your eyebrows grow, making sure all the areas you want to remove have wax. Remember, only apply it to the hairs you want to remove.

5. Cover your eyebrow with the muslin cloth strip in the direction of your eyebrow growth; a part of the strip should be left free of hair so that you can use it for removal. Firmly press the strip in the direction your eyebrow grows several times to ensure it is attached, and let it cool slightly.

6. Grasp the part of the cloth strip that extends beyond the eyebrow and, holding your eyebrow skin taut with your other hand, remove the strip with one quick pull in the opposite direction to the hair growth (*not* upwards). If any hairs are remaining, put the strip back on and pull it off again.

7. Clean any remaining wax off your skin using baby oil or a wax remover.

8. Finish by applying aloe vera to reduce redness.

FILLING IN BROWS

Think of this step as creating a shadow behind the brows.

To do this, use a shade lighter than your brow colour and fill in. If your eyebrows are very fair, choose a colour a shade or two darker than your brows. While many companies have developed products for shading your eyebrows, it's really quite simple to do yourself. Let's take a look.

TOOLS FOR FILLING IN

The following are tools you can use when shaping your brows. Pencils are a great tool when you need to lengthen or fill in a weak brow, while eye shadows are used to add more colour and fullness to a brow. You can use each separately or both together, depending on your need.

Eyebrow pencil: You can use the point of an eyebrow pencil to lightly draw in hairs for a natural look, or shade in the brows for a more dramatic look. There are five shades typically used to fill brows; each is matched to a particular hair colour:

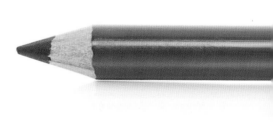

> **Taupe:** Blonde and red hair
>
> **Light brown:** Dark blonde and light brown hair
>
> **Medium brown:** Light to medium brown hair
>
> **Dark brown:** Medium to dark brown hair
>
> **Black:** Black hair and dark skin

Eye shadow: You can use a matte eye shadow with an angle brush to fill in and shape your brows. Again, I suggest you use the shade that corresponds with your hair colour:

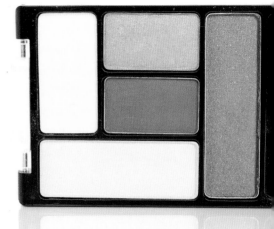

> **Taupe:** Blonde hair
>
> **Light brown:** Light to medium brown hair
>
> **Dark brown:** Dark brown hair
>
> **Black:** Black hair

BASIC BROW FILLING

Ultimately, your goal is to give the illusion of a fuller natural brow. The following walks you step by step through how to do this. Refer back to "The Perfect Eyebrow" for a refresher on the three points of the brow.

1. Point 1 should be the darkest and fullest area of the eyebrow. Use the tip of your pencil and begin by drawing a line vertical to the nose.

2. Lightly draw the bottom line of the brow from the starting point, over the arch, and down to point 3.

3. Lightly create a parallel line at the top of the brow you are creating.

4. Use a lighter touch as you move from point 2 to point 3 to give a softer finish to the brow. The brow should become thinner as you get to point 3.

5. Lightly fill in between the two lines. Remember, the brow should be darker between points 1 and 2 and become gradually lighter as you move towards point 3.

6. You can use a disposable mascara wand to brush over the eyebrow you've created. This softens the lines and blends them into your natural eyebrows.

What You Need

EYEBROW PENCIL

MASCARA WAND

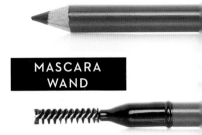

Creating an Eyelift

For an instant eyelift, apply soft white eye shadow above your eyebrow and soft pink eye shadow below the arch of your eyebrow. This will define and elevate it.

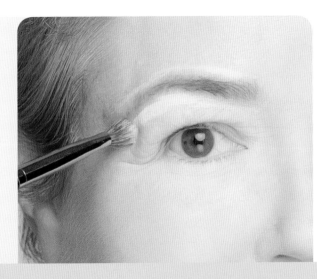

Creating a Brow Stencil

To simplify filling in your eyebrows, you can create a brow stencil, using the following items.

Vellum paper or tracing paper

Craft knife

Cutting mat

HB pencil

Hold the vellum or tracing paper to your eyebrow and lightly trace your eyebrow, using the eyebrow shape as a guide.

Choose the eyebrow shape you would like to create: round, angled, soft angled, curved, or flat. Sketch the shape over the brow you traced on the vellum paper. Erase the parts of the old brow you don't want and then, using the craft knife, cut the resulting brow shape out of the paper. Use the point of your knife to carefully trim the inside of the stencil.

If you would like a stencil for each brow, turn the stencil upside down and trace a mirror image of the brow. Using the craft knife, cut out the second brow stencil. Label one stencil R (right) and the other L (left).

Place the stencil over your eyebrow and colour in with the appropriate eyebrow pencil or matte eye shadow. If you are using only one stencil, turn the stencil over and place it on the opposite brow; otherwise, use the second stencil.

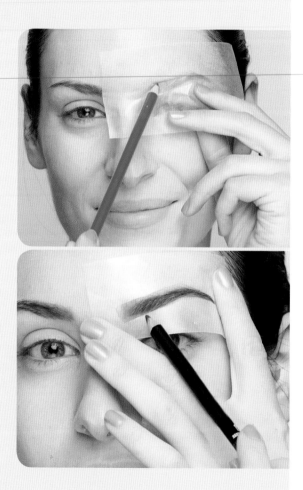

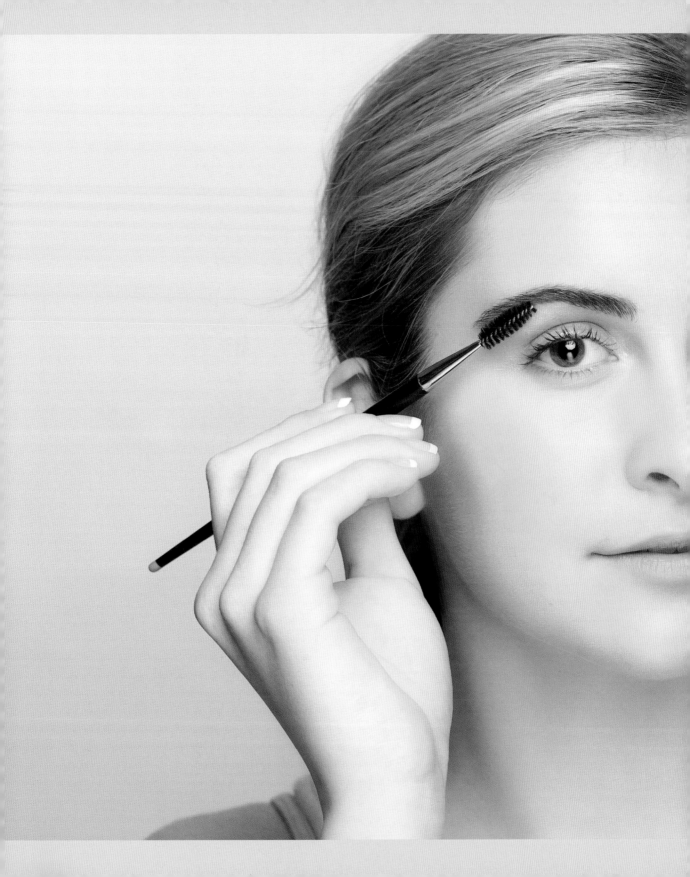

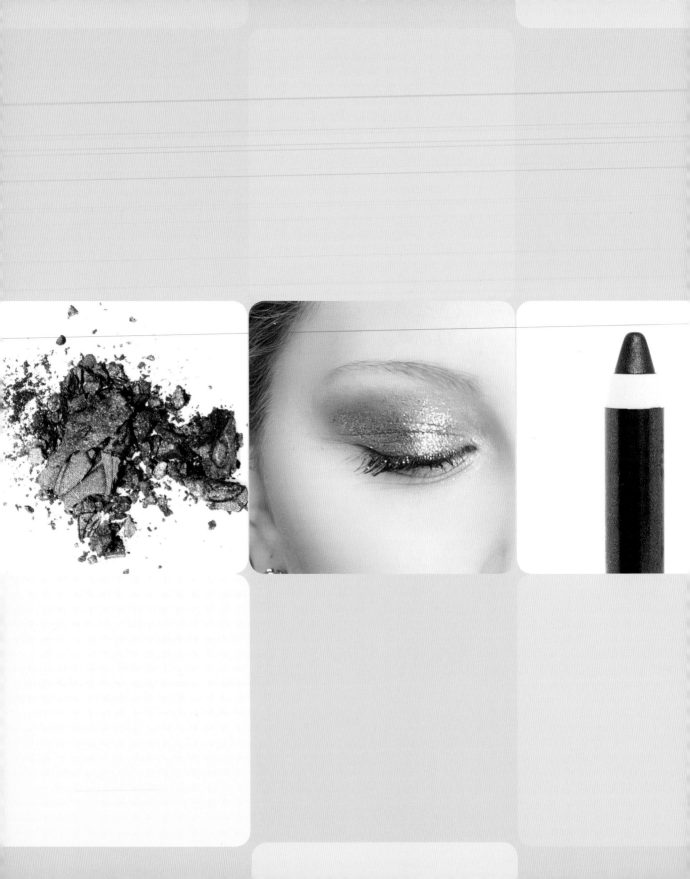

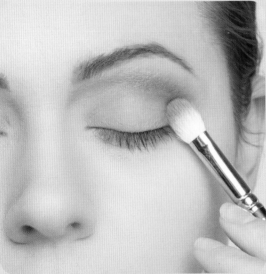

CHAPTER 11
EYES

The eyes are your most important feature. But with so much variety on offer, choosing the right eye shadow product in the right colour can seem incredibly intimidating. And that's before considering eyeliner, mascara, eyelash curlers, or false eyelashes.

In this chapter, I help you choose the appropriate eye shadow, eyeliner, and lash treatment. I also give you plenty of tips to make your eyes look their most dazzling, whatever your eye shape.

TYPES OF EYE SHADOW

There are thousands of eye shadow pigments (or colours).

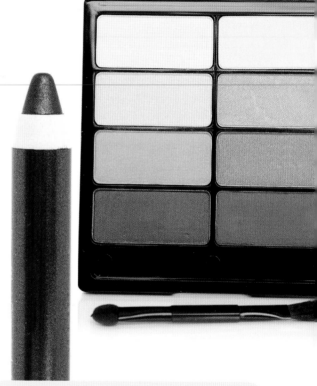

Eye shadows come in the following forms: pressed powder, loose powder, cream, and mineral.

Pressed powder: Eye shadow in pressed form comes in a compact, which makes it easy to carry. You can apply pressed powder with a brush, a sponge applicator, or an applicator supplied with the shadow.

Loose powder: Eye shadow in loose form comes in a shaker. This type of eye shadow is applied with a brush. Loose powder allows a stronger application of pigment for a bolder eye look.

Cream: This comes in a variety of colours and provides more coverage due to its thicker consistency. However, because it is a cream, it can easily crease; therefore, I don't recommend cream shadow for mature eyes.

Mineral: This eye shadow is great alternative to other shadow types. It comes in some beautiful colours and is great for sensitive skin, as it doesn't irritate.

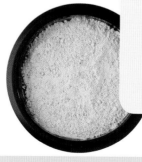

Setting Your Eye Shadow

For longer wear, use cream shadow as a primer for a pressed or loose eye shadow in the same colour. You can then apply the powder shadow to set the cream.

EYE SHADOW FINISHES

Another difference between eye shadows is the type of finish they have: sheer, matte, shimmer, metallic, or glitter.

Sheer: These eye shadows have a light pigment. They provide a hint of colour and are great to use for everyday natural looks.

Matte: Shadows that do not have a shine or reflect light offer a matte finish. Matte shadows are often beautiful, silky colours that are used for natural looks. They are great for mature eyes, since they do not highlight the fine lines associated with ageing.

Shimmer: These types of eye shadow contain light-reflecting materials that provide their shimmer finish, giving depth and interest to the colours. In addition, you can easily blend shades in this finish to create a striking look.

Metallic: These eye shadows are similar to a shimmer shadow in terms of finish. They typically come in shades the colour of metal (gold, silver, copper, and dark grey). Metallic finishes create a dramatic evening look and are great on darker skin.

Glitter: Cosmetic glitter is ground more finely than craft glitter and gives a sparkle to eye shadows. A glitter finish creates a theatrical eye effect and is typically worn by teenage girls. Because glitter is loose and can shed easily, it should be the last thing you apply when doing your make-up.

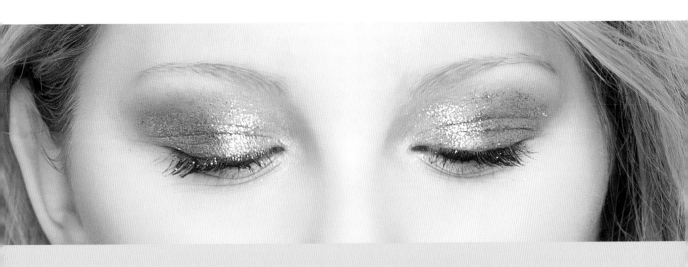

CHOOSING AN EYE SHADOW COLOUR

You may be wondering, "How do I choose a colour that looks best on me?"

Any good make-up artist will tell you it's important to first have an understanding of the colour wheel. So before you pick out eye shadow, let's review the colour wheel and the relationship between primary, secondary, and tertiary colours.

All colours derive from the *primary colours*: red, yellow, and blue. Primary colours cannot be produced by mixing other colours. *Secondary colours* are a combination of two primary colours, resulting in orange, green, or violet, depending on the colours combined. *Tertiary colours* are a combination of a primary and a secondary colour. For example, red-orange, red-violet, yellow-orange, yellow-green, blue-violet, and blue-green are tertiary colours.

All colours have complementary colours, which are colours that lie opposite each other on the colour wheel. When combined in the right proportions, these pairs will create white or black. Here are some common examples:

- Red is complementary to the colour green.

- Blue is complementary to the colour orange.

- Yellow is complementary to the colour violet.

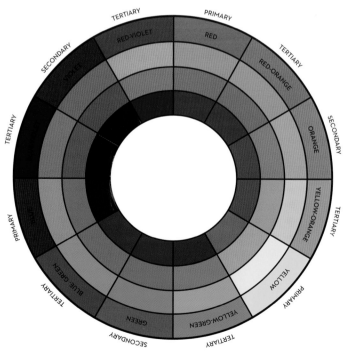

Now that you understand the colour wheel, a good rule of thumb is to use your eye colour to help choose the appropriate colour for eye shadow. Here are the shades I recommend based on eye colour.

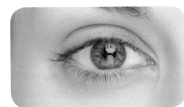

Blue eyes: The complementary colour to blue is orange. Therefore, look for colours that have shades of orange, such as gold, copper, apricot, and peach.

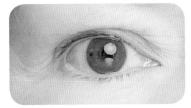

Green eyes: The complementary colour to green is red. So look for eye shadow in shades of red, such as plum and wine.

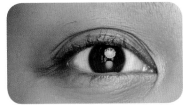

Brown eyes: Brown is a neutral colour, so any eye shadow colour will work with it. Typically, blue and purple colours make brown eyes stand out.

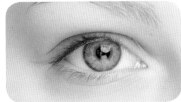

Hazel eyes: People with hazel eyes can enjoy a wide spectrum of shadow colours, due to their flecked hues. This eye colour can handle many different shades of eye make-up. However, blue is one exception – it can make hazel eyes look greyish.

Salvaging a Broken Eye Shadow

Did you drop your eye shadow? No problem! Here are a couple of ways you can salvage it:

- If you want to still use it as a shadow, add a few drops of surgical spirit to the broken shadow. You can then press it back together with a coin, reshaping and remixing the shadow.

- For something different, take the eye shadow and mix it with a clear nail polish. You have now created some great nail polish!

APPLYING EYE SHADOW

Once you've chosen the appropriate colours for your skin tone, eye colour, and eye shadow design, it's time to apply them.

Basic shadow placement begins with putting on three eye shadow colours: light, medium, and dark. You then proceed to blend the eye shadow colours into one another; this softens any harsh lines between colours. For the best outcome, the entire lid should be covered in make-up. Leaving any part of the lid exposed can weaken the overall look.

What You Need

EYE SHADOW BRUSH

LIGHT EYE SHADOW

DARK EYE SHADOW

MEDIUM EYE SHADOW

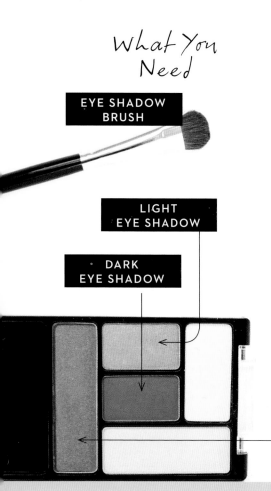

1. Apply the medium eye shadow colour on your eyelid. This colour is typically the predominant colour (for example, gold) and is the statement colour in the palette.

2. Apply the dark eye shadow colour in the crease of your eye; these are usually made up of shades of brown or black. This is a form of contouring that creates definition for the eye.

3. Apply the light eye shadow colour from the crease to just under the eyebrow and from the brow bone into the tear duct. This is a white, ivory, or cream colour used to highlight the eye.

4. Using your eye shadow brush, blend the darkest colour just into the highlight colour, moving back and forth like a windscreen wiper. Repeat the blending into the medium eye shadow colour. Remember to only blend where a colour meets a colour; pulling a colour completely into another will make the application appear sloppy and muddy.

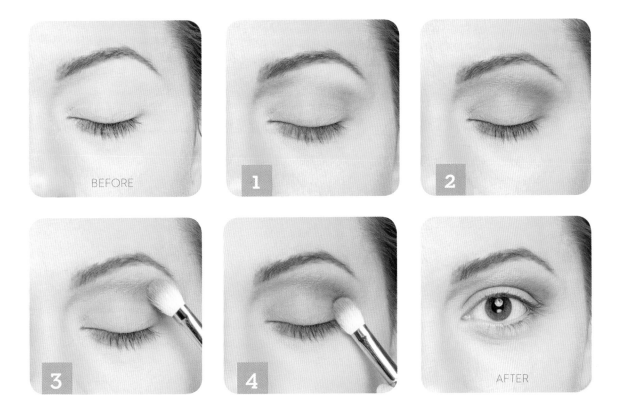

BEFORE

1

2

3

4

AFTER

Making Colours Pop

Want to make coloured eye shadows pop? First, apply a white eye cream to the eyelid, and then dab your favourite eye shadow colour on top. The white eye cream will intensify the coloured eye shadow.

TYPES OF EYELINER

Originally introduced by the ancient Egyptians and gaining popularity in the 1920s, eyeliner has long been used as a tool to accentuate the eyes.

While the first eyeliner was made from kohl (lead sulphide), manufacturers have since created eyeliner with much safer ingredients. You can find eyeliner in pencil, liquid, gel pot, and eye shadow form.

Pencil: Eyeliner pencils come in shades varying from white to black, are easy to apply, and are very affordable. You can buy pencils in thin and jumbo sizes, depending on how thick you want the line to be. Typically, pencils will require the use of a cosmetic pencil sharpener. Eyeliner pencils are particularly great to use for smoky eye applications because of the ease with which you can smudge them.

Liquid: This eyeliner goes on wet and provides a stronger colour pigment than pencil. It also comes with a pen tip, which makes application much easier. Liquid liner requires a steady hand, but it's worth the effort when it comes to a clean look. Because liquid liner needs a moment to dry, I suggest keeping your eye closed for a few seconds; otherwise, smudging may occur.

Gel pot: Gel eyeliner comes in a small pot and is applied with an angle brush. Like liquid eyeliner, gel eyeliner has a strong pigment; however, you can smudge the product into place before it sets.

Eye shadow: You can also use eye shadow as a liner. In fact, I encourage you to use a matte eye shadow with a make-up brush prior to using a pencil or pen. If you are making a cat eye, you can lay down the eye shadow as a guide for your liner. Additionally, eye shadow is great as an eyeliner for oily skin because it absorbs the oil, allowing the shadow to stay on the lid.

BASIC EYELINER APPLICATION

The following are the basic steps for applying eyeliner.

Remember, you should begin your eyeliner application only after you have finished applying your eye shadow.

1. Place your index finger at the crease of your eye and gently lift the eyelid. This is especially important if you have a heavy-fold eyelid or mature skin that has lost some of its elasticity.

2. Beginning at the last eyelash located closest to your tear duct, start drawing a line following the natural lash line. This may take a few strokes of the liner.

3. Stop at the end of your outer eye, being careful not to go past the eyelashes.

4. Repeat steps 2 and 3 on the lower lash line. For a natural look, start at the centre of the eye and work to the outside corner. Blend at the centre to create a soft line.

GOING BEYOND BASIC: EYELINER BY ERA

Looking for something beyond a basic line?

Different eras have provided looks that are fun and easy to copy. The following take you through the popular eyeliner styles of several decades, suggesting the best eyeliner products to achieve them.

1920S

The 1920s was the period that launched the smoky look of eyeliner with a kohl effect. To create the 1920s smoky eye, take your eyeliner pencil or gel pot and follow the natural curve of the lash line, tracing all around the eye. Finally, smudge outside the lower lash line; this creates a softer (smoky) effect with the liner.

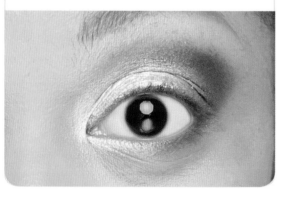

1940S

The 1940s emphasized liner on top of the lid. To create this look, take your eyeliner pencil or liquid liner along the top lash line, following the curve of the eye with a thick line. On the bottom lash line, use an eye shadow or pencil to create a thin line, stopping before your tear duct.

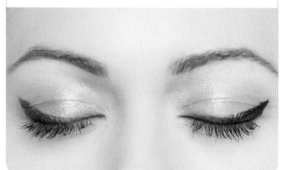

1950S AND 1960S

The cat eye trend began in the 1950s and became overexaggerated in the 1960s as outrageous fashion styles exploded. To create this bold eye, take a liquid or gel eyeliner and draw a thick black line on the top lash line. When you approach the outer edge, swoop the liner upwards.

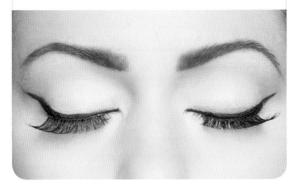

1970S

In the 1970s, eyeliner switched to a more natural look composed of browns and whites. To create this look, use a brown eyeliner and follow the natural curve of your lash line. Apply to the top only.

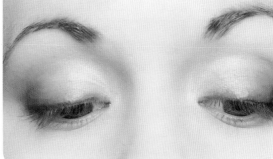

1980S

This style allows you to use any colour eyeliner to complete your look, though black will be the most dramatic. To copy this look, take any liner type and line completely around the entire eye and into the water line – in fact, the more severe and dramatic the eyeliner, the better.

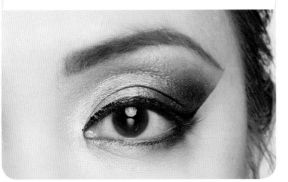

Polishing Your Eye Look

To give your make-up application a more polished look, take the primary eye shadow colour used on your eyelid and apply the same colour along your bottom lash line using an angle brush. For example, if you used a turquoise eye shadow, use the same colour in the tear duct area to marry the look together.

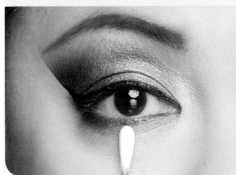

PARTS OF THE EYE AND THEIR ROLE IN MAKE-UP

With full eye make-up, the entire eye must be considered. Each part should be addressed during a make-up application.

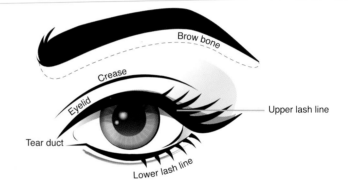

- **Brow bone:** Found directly under the eyebrow, the highlight colour is applied to this section.

- **Crease:** Found at the top of the lid and the beginning of the brow bone, it is the section where the skin rolls into the eye socket. Depending on the brow bone, the crease can be deep set to nonexistent.

- **Eyelid:** The half-moon-shaped section of skin between the upper lash line and the crease, this is the primary space for eye shadow.

- **Upper lash line:** Found along the edge of the lid closest to the eye, this is where eyeliner, mascara, and false eyelashes are used.

- **Tear duct:** Also known as the *inner eye*, this is found at the corner of the eye closest to the nose. Liner and shadow can be applied in this section.

- **Lower lash line:** Found at the bottom of the eye, this is another place to use eyeliner and mascara.

CORRECTING YOUR EYE SHAPE WITH FULL EYE MAKE-UP

Now that you know the parts of the eye, it's time go over the 10 eye shapes – almond, wide set, close set, deep set, prominent, small, monolid, hooded, upturned, and downturned – and how to correct them, if necessary, to create a balanced look.

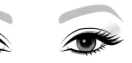

ALMOND (AVERAGE) EYES

This is the shape you want to replicate. The almond eye shape is the most balanced in width and height and has equal distance from the upper lash line to the crease and the crease to the brow bone. If you have this eye shape, you will find it easy to create most eye make-up looks, whatever the technique.

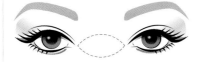

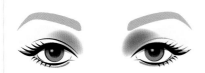

WIDE-SET EYES

Wide-set eyes are set more than an eye width apart. The goal of your eye make-up application should be to bring the eyes in towards the nose. Apply darker eye shadow colours in the corners of the eyes. This technique draws the eyes in towards the nose.

Eye shadow colours and placement can assist in bringing wide-set eyes inwards. Use light eye shadow colours on the middle to outside eyes and darker eye shadow colours closer to the nose to draw focus inwards. If you choose to wear dark eye shadows, do not apply past the end of the eyebrow; this accentuates the wideness of the eyes.

CLOSE-SET EYES

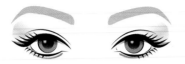

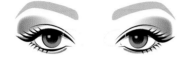

Close-set eyes are set less than an eye width apart. Therefore, you want to use your eye make-up to create space between the eyes.

The trick is to create more space between the bridge of the nose and the corners of the eyes. This is achieved by placing a light colour, such as white or off-white, at the inside corners of the eyes.

DEEP-SET EYES

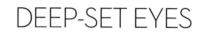

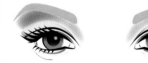

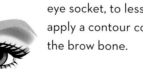

Deep-set eyes have protruding eye sockets. Because the eyes are set further back into the eye socket, they create shadows. The aim is to reduce the shadows the eye sockets cast onto the eyelids.

Apply a light eye shadow on the eyelid, blending it into the eye socket, to lessen the shadows. To finish the application, apply a contour colour in the crease and blend up and over the brow bone.

PROMINENT EYES

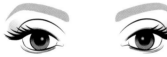

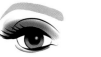

Prominent eyes are large, round eyes where more of the white of the eyes can be seen. Your goal is to create the illusion that the eyes are smaller.

Bring your darker eye shadow closer to the top lash lines. Follow this with a heavy, dark eyeliner on the top lash line. Finish the application by adding the dark eyeliner to the water lines (the pink area behind your lower lashes) to give the illusion of smaller eyes.

SMALL EYES

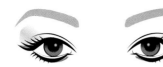

Small eyes have less space between the lash lines, with very little of the whites of the eyes showing. The goal is to make the eyes look bigger and more pronounced.

Apply a white pencil along the lower lash lines. Apply darker eyeliner just below the white eyeliner. This technique gives the illusion of a larger eye shape.

MONOLID EYES

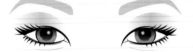

Monolid eyes have little to no crease in the eyelids and no brow bone. There is a fairly flat surface between the eyelid and the eyebrow and a larger surface area to play with. Because there is a minimal crease in the eyelid, the goal is to create one.

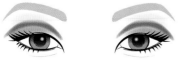

Apply the contour (darkest) shadow in a half-moon shape where you imagine a crease to be on each eye. Blend your medium shadow on the creases. Finally, apply the highlight eye shadow.

HOODED EYES

Hooded eyes have heavy folds of skin that hang over the eye sockets, which are more prominent in mature skin. The trick is to create a contour on the lids.

Sweep a matte contour colour close to the lash lines. Next, layer your medium eye shadow colour above the contour, and blend highlight (light eye shadow) from the corner of the eyes upwards onto the brow bones. This reduces the apparent weight in the eyelids.

Lastly, apply eyeliner to the upper lash lines. Remember, the lids are covering a lot of the eyes. Therefore, be careful not to make the liner too thick, as it will get lost in the folds.

UPTURNED EYES

Upturned eyes angle upwards at the outer corners of the eyes. As an example, most Disney princesses are drawn with upturned eyes! To minimize the amount of angle, imagine the eyelids are divided in half.

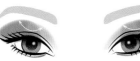

Apply a medium shadow from the centre and blend downwards towards the tear ducts. Apply the contour (darkest) colour from the middle of the eyes towards the outer corners. Finish by blending the colour in a "U" shape (not following the upwards slope). This angles the eyes downwards, creating the illusion that the eyes aren't so upturned.

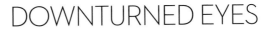

DOWNTURNED EYES

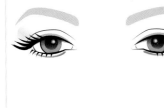

Downturned eyes angle downwards at the outer corners. To correct this, you want to give the eyes a lift.

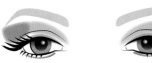

Apply a medium shadow from the tear ducts to just beyond the middle of the eyes. Apply a contour colour just past the middle of the eyes, sweeping it upwards at the outer corners. This creates the lift you need.

TYPES OF MASCARA

Mascara is a cosmetic formulated with pigments, waxes, oils, and preservatives to darken and thicken the eyelashes.

Just like the hair on your head, eyelashes can be thin, brittle, and unruly. Therefore, different types of mascara have been designed to address these common issues.

Waterproof mascara: This type is formulated with mineral oils and waxes that enable it to stay on your eyelashes through water, tears, and sweat.

Volumizing mascara: The formula for this mascara contains silicone polymers and thickening agents, which give the illusion of thicker eyelashes.

Smudge-proof mascara: Formulated with a wax-oil base, this mascara is great for people who are very active and don't want to retouch their mascara during the day.

Curling mascara: This type is a bit thicker than regular mascara. It comes with a wand designed to curl the lashes.

Lengthening mascara: This mascara contains tiny synthetic fibres that cling to one another and to the lash, giving the appearance of longer lashes.

Lash-defining mascara: This provides a combination of volumizing, lengthening, and colour to your eyelashes. Often waterproof, it's considered an all-in-one mascara.

Eyelash primer: This is good if you wear make-up every day, as it coats the lashes, protecting them against damage from daily mascara use. Primer also provides moisture to dry lashes and acts as an undercoat so your mascara goes on evenly.

Defining Your Lashes

Use an eyeliner pen to highlight your bottom eyelashes. While it does take some time, you can define each lash individually, making them stand out.

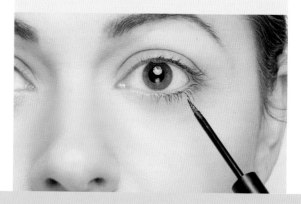

MASCARA COLOURS

You can choose mascara in a variety of colours, depending on your needs.

Black: Black mascara is great for a dramatic and bold look, and for use on darker skin tones.

Brown: Brown mascara is a bit softer than black mascara and works for natural daytime looks. It's a good colour choice for people with very fair skin.

Fashion colours: This refers to colours beyond the typical black and brown, such as blue, yellow, and green. Fashion-colour mascara helps enhance a dramatic, youthful look.

Clear: If you already have thick, full eyelashes and just want definition, try a clear mascara. It simply provides shine and separation for your lashes.

Mascara Application Tips

Have you ever applied your mascara perfectly, only to blink and have it stain and smudge? To avoid smudges on the skin beneath your lashes, lay a plastic spoon under your bottom lashes, and then apply your mascara. If you're looking to keep your upper lashes and eye make-up pristine, hold an index card behind the top lashes when applying your mascara.

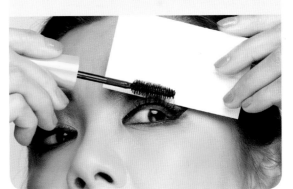

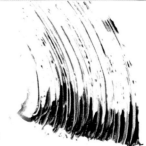

MASCARA WANDS

You might not realize it, but the proper mascara wand is just as important as the mascara itself.

The following are the different types of mascara wand you can find, along with the specific lash issues they address.

Short wand: A mascara wand with short bristles is great for short eyelashes.

Long wand: This type of wand has evenly spaced bristles that are ideal for lengthening your lashes.

Round wand: A round wand with dense bristles can help give volume to your lashes.

Spherical brush wand: This type of wand, with bristles on a sphere, is designed for individual eyelash application. While using this is more time consuming, you'll end up with well-defined lashes.

Curved wand: This wand has evenly spaced bristles that lift and curl your eyelashes.

Cleaning Off Excess Mascara

Do you always have too much product on your mascara wand? Wipe a little off on a tissue before applying. Pay close attention to the end of the wand, where mascara tends to gather and clump.

Recycling Your Wands

Looking to save some money? Keep your favourite wands from expensive discarded mascaras, clean them, and use them to achieve a better application with less expensive mascaras.

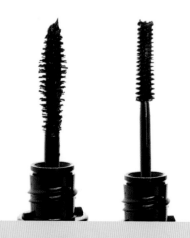

BASIC MASCARA APPLICATION

Applying mascara does not have to be difficult.

The basic rule of thumb is to apply to your top lashes only, unless you want your eyes to look more open. The following walks you through how to get the best mascara coverage for your lashes.

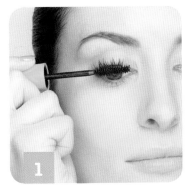 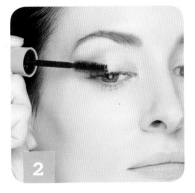 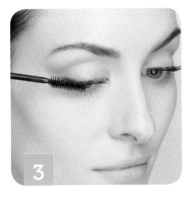

1. Place the mascara wand deep into the base of the lashes, wiggling it in, left to right. You want to have good coverage near the roots, as it is mascara in this area – not at the tips – that gives the illusion of length.

2. Pull the wand up and through the lashes, wiggling as you go. This wiggling helps separate the lashes.

3. Close your eye and place the mascara wand on top of the lashes at the base. Pull the wand through to remove any clumps.

Declumping Your Mascara

Are you trying to declump your mascara? Do not pump the wand into the mascara. This incorporates air into the product and dries it out. Instead, swirl the wand in the tube. If the mascara begins to get clumpy and swirling doesn't help, add a few eye drops to it. This will refresh the mascara.

OTHER EYELASH TOOLS AND TECHNIQUES

A couple of coats of mascara isn't the only thing that can improve the look of your lashes.

The following tools and techniques help you achieve beautiful eyelashes beyond the mascara tube.

EYELASH CURLER

An eyelash curler is a tool used to curl your upper eyelashes prior to applying mascara or false eyelashes. It's normally made out of metal and has rubber strips on the curlers where the lashes are gripped. While using it is a fairly simple process, the following step-by-step shows you how to get the best results from your eyelash curler.

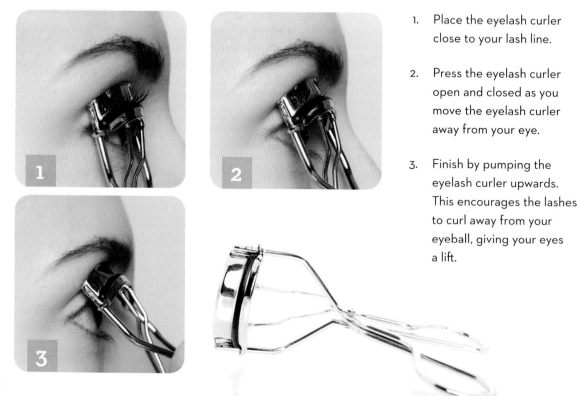

1. Place the eyelash curler close to your lash line.

2. Press the eyelash curler open and closed as you move the eyelash curler away from your eye.

3. Finish by pumping the eyelash curler upwards. This encourages the lashes to curl away from your eyeball, giving your eyes a lift.

Longer-Lasting Curled Lashes

For longer-lasting curled lashes, try heating your eyelash curler with a hairdryer for five seconds before use. The heat will curl your lashes just like curling tongs curl hair. However, be careful not to overheat the tool, or you'll risk burning your lashes and delicate eyelids.

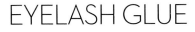

EYELASH GLUE

Eyelash glue is a cosmetic adhesive that comes in white or black colours and is used to apply false eyelashes. In most cases, the glue dries clear after application. This glue is safe to use near your eyes and peels off quite easily.

FALSE EYELASHES

A make-up staple between 1920 and 1960, false eyelashes were once a must in every woman's make-up arsenal. However, that trend came to a halt during the relaxed 1970s, when the natural look became popular. Today, false eyelashes are still a great choice when you want to glam up your look.

There are two types of false lashes: strip and individual lashes. Made with human hair or synthetic materials, they come in many styles, colours, and lengths and are applied with eyelash glue. While they are not designed to be worn when showering, sleeping, or swimming, they can be used to add some drama, day or night.

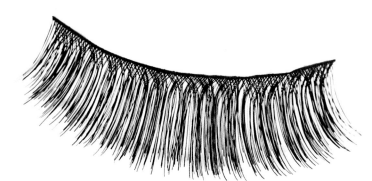

STRIP EYELASHES

Strip lashes come on a strip or band in different lengths and colours. If cared for properly, strip lashes can be reused.

The following step-by-step guide assures a quick and clean application. While I use a bobby pin (or kirby grip) to press the lashes down, feel free to use tweezers or the end of your make-up brush. When you're ready to remove them, gently pull them off; you can use a gentle cleanser to remove any remaining glue.

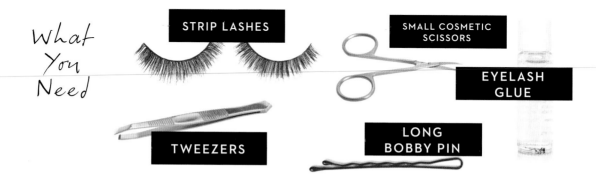

What You Need

STRIP LASHES

SMALL COSMETIC SCISSORS

EYELASH GLUE

TWEEZERS

LONG BOBBY PIN

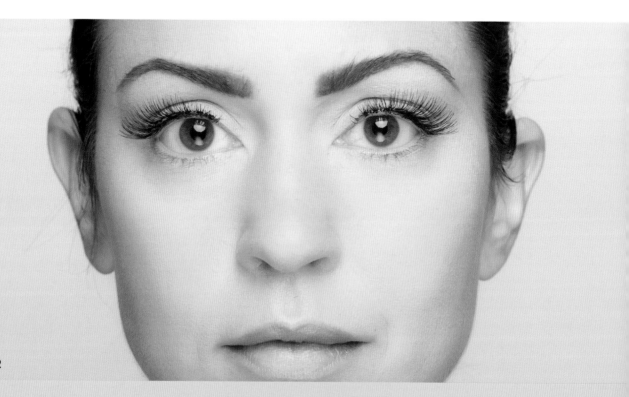

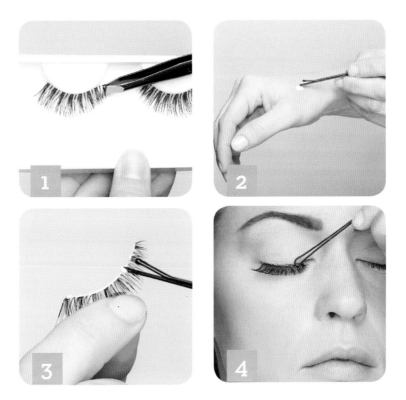

1. With a pair of tweezers, remove a false eyelash strip from its container. If the strip is too long, trim from the outside (wider) part of the lash strip.

2. Put a drop of eyelash glue on one end of the bobby pin.

3. Apply a thin line of glue to the eyelash with the bobby pin, and let the glue air-dry for about 30 seconds. If the glue is too wet, the strip will slide around.

4. Lay the strip as close to the lash line as possible. Press the strip lash down with the clean side of the bobby pin. Continue pressing the lash down in the centre and work left to right until the lash has adhered.

Eyelash Extensions

If you want permanently full and long lashes, consider looking into eyelash extensions. These consist of sections of at least three false eyelashes glued together. Unlike temporary false eyelashes, eyelash extensions aren't damaged by water from showering or swimming, making them a great option if you enjoy an active lifestyle. This lash type also gives you much more control in terms of how thick you want your lashes and where you put them.

Eyelash extensions come in three types: synthetic, mink, and silk. Whatever type you choose, they have to be applied by a professional. Extension lashes are permanent, not reusable, and can last up to six or eight weeks. Because extension eyelashes fall out when you lose your natural lashes, it is recommended you get a touch-up every three to four weeks.

INDIVIDUAL EYELASHES

Unlike strip lashes, individual eyelashes typically come as one single lash or in a group of three lashes. They are used to fill in lashes where needed and can create a more natural look than strip lashes. The following takes you through how to apply them.

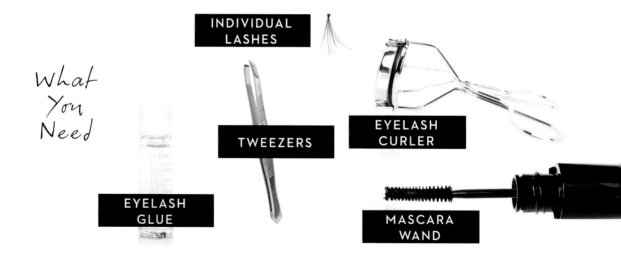

What You Need

INDIVIDUAL LASHES

TWEEZERS

EYELASH CURLER

EYELASH GLUE

MASCARA WAND

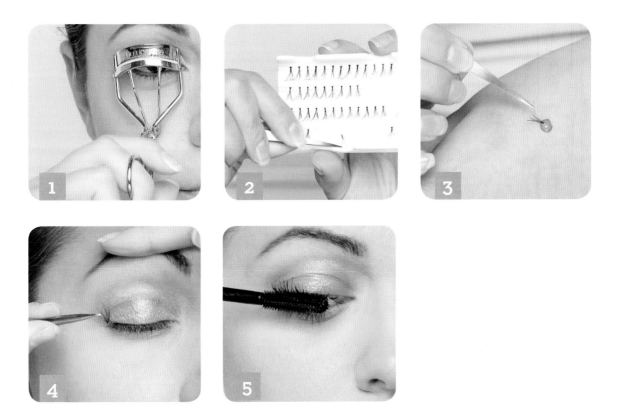

1. Curl your natural lashes to give them some bend. This will make it easier to hide the fake lashes among them. Also, prep your lashes with one coat of mascara. This also helps the lashes blend more seamlessly with the false lashes.

2. Using a clean set of tweezers or your fingers, grab one lash from your set of individual lashes.

3. Lightly dip the end of the lash into a dot of eyelash glue.

4. Starting from the outside of your eye, apply the lash right into your lash line using the tweezers. Let dry for a few seconds if you landed in the right spot, or take your time moving it so the eyelash lines up with your natural lashes. Continue to fill in as many lashes as you need.

5. After you have applied the lashes and allowed the glue to set and dry for a few minutes, gently comb through your lashes with a mascara wand. This ensures the false and natural lashes aren't all poking out in different directions.

OTHER EYELASH TOOLS AND TECHNIQUES

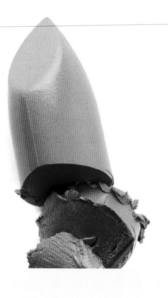
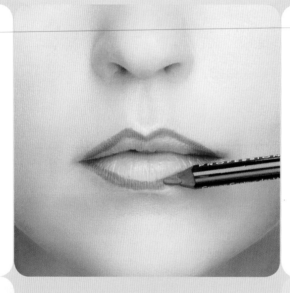

CHAPTER 12
LIPS

The lips are the second most important feature next to the eyes. Throughout the decades, there have been full red, hot pink, nude glossy, and soft dusty rose lip trends. Today, the market offers dozens of different shades of lip colour. Taking the time to master the techniques for a great lip application lets you add the finishing touch to a flawless look.

In this chapter, I discuss lip colour products and how to choose the right lip colour. I also talk about applying lip liner and correcting your lip shape to balance your face.

LIP COLOUR PRODUCTS

Lip colour products come in pencils, lipsticks, lip stains, and lip glosses.

Each type has its uses and advantages. Take a look at each type and see which you might want to add to your make-up arsenal.

Lip pencil: This comes in a variety of shades and, like any cosmetic pencil, must be sharpened with a cosmetic pencil sharpener to keep its point. A lip pencil is not only great for outline work, but also for filling the lips to act as a base colour.

Lipstick: This is the most common lip colour application. It has a creamy consistency, is made from various forms of wax, and can contain emollients and oils for soft, healthy lips. Lipstick in tube form allows you to apply your lip colour without any additional tools. However, cream lipstick, which comes in a pot or palette, requires a lip brush for application.

Fixing a Broken Lipstick

Oops! Did you break your lipstick? Not to worry! Take a lighter or match (being careful not to burn yourself) and melt one end of the stick. Next, reattach the stick and hold it in place until it hardens. Your lipstick should be as good as new!

The Secret to Long-Lasting Lip Colour

Looking for lip colour with staying power? Using a lip pencil as a base colour, line your lips and fill them in with the lip pencil. Next, apply a layer of lipstick and set with a matching powder eye shadow.

Lip stain: Made from a water and gel formula, this has a high pigment content and can last up to 18 hours. Lip stain is more difficult to remove than lipstick or lip pencil, requiring you to use a make-up remover for the best results.

Lip gloss: This comes in a gel consistency and is great for hydrating lips. Gloss comes in many complementary shades to lipstick, making it ideal to apply on top of matte lipstick for a juicy finish. Dabbing clear or tinted gloss in the centre of the lip can also help create the illusion of fullness.

Lip balm: Created to help repair cracked and chapped lips and to add moisture, lip balm is made with wax or paraffin and can contain flavours, pigments, and even sunscreen. Applying lip balm before applying lipstick will help your lipstick go on more smoothly.

Setting Your Lipstick

To set your lipstick, take a single-ply tissue and lay it across your finished lips. Apply setting powder to a brush, and then swipe the setting powder over the tissue. The powder will set your lips through the tissue.

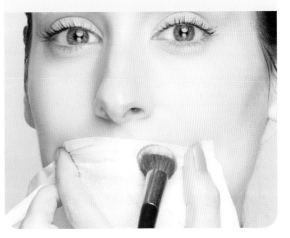

Getting to the Last of Your Gloss

Many have dealt with the headache of being at the end of their lip gloss tube and unable to get the rest of the product out. However, you don't have to consign it to the bin. Dipping the tube into hot water will loosen up the product so you can access it.

Creating Your Own Lipstick Palette

With the following tools, you can create your own lipstick palette from lipsticks that are currently in separate containers.

Two different lipstick tubes

Large metal spoon

Candle

Empty and clean contact lens case

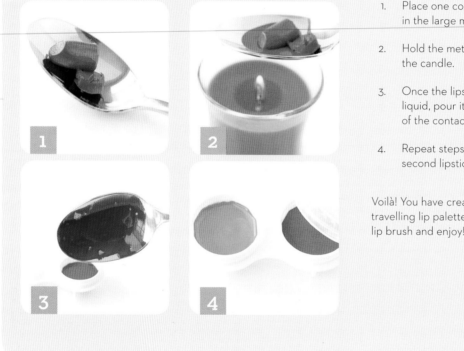

1. Place one colour of lipstick in the large metal spoon.

2. Hold the metal spoon over the candle.

3. Once the lipstick becomes liquid, pour it into one side of the contact lens case.

4. Repeat steps 1 to 3 with the second lipstick.

Voilà! You have created your own travelling lip palette. Apply with a lip brush and enjoy!

CHOOSING THE RIGHT LIP COLOUR

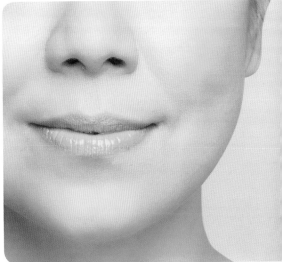

Beauty product shelves are filled with numerous shades of lip colour.

How do you choose the right shade? One rule of thumb is to choose a lip colour that is complementary to your cheek colour; you don't want your lip and cheek colours to jar.

Another consideration is your skin tone. You want a shade that doesn't wash you out or age you. The following are the best colours for different skin tones.

SKIN TONE	LIP COLOR		
FAIR	LIGHT PINK	LIGHT PEACH	
	BEIGE	GOLDEN BROWN	
MEDIUM	MEDIUM PINK	RED	
	ORANGEY PEACH	APRICOT	
OLIVE	DARK ROSE	DARK RED	
	BERRY	DARK APRICOT	
DARK	BROWNISH RED	DARK FUCHSIA	
	DARK BERRY	GOLDEN BEIGE	

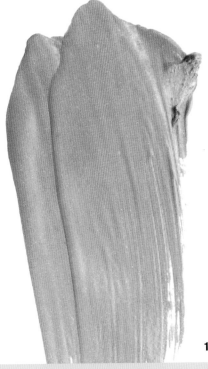

APPLYING LIP LINER

Are you having trouble lining your lips?

Do you simply need a process that's fast and easy? Follow these steps to get beautifully lined lips in no time!

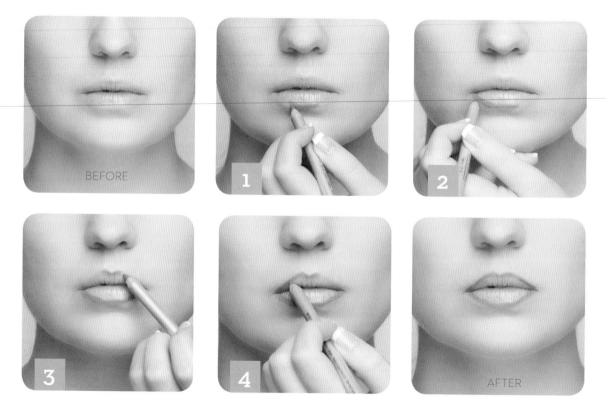

BEFORE   1   2
3   4   AFTER

1. With your lip pencil, create a U shape at the centre of the bottom lip.

2. Starting at one outside corner of the bottom lip, follow the lip line down to meet the centre line. Repeat from the other outside corner.

3. On the upper lip, create a V shape within the cupid's bow.

4. Position your lip pencil at the corner of the mouth and travel up the lip, curving over and into the V. Repeat on the other side.

CREATING BALANCE BASED ON YOUR LIP SHAPE

Lips come in all shapes and sizes, but they basically boil down to these four types: average, wide, thin, and combination.

The goal of your make-up application is to ensure your lips are in proportion to your face. Sometimes, to create balance, you may need to correct your lip shape. The following shows you how to do this for each lip shape, using foundation, lip pencil (sharpened, of course), and lip colour or lip gloss.

AVERAGE

With average lips, the top and bottom lips are equal in size. In addition, the outer edges of the mouth align with the pupils of the eyes. Because the mouth is in proportion to the face, the lips need no correction. Therefore, simply apply your lip pencil and/or colour by following the natural lip.

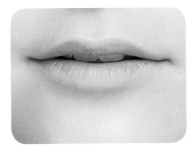

WIDE

With wide lips, the top and bottom lips are full and therefore too big for the face shape. The goal is to reduce the fullness of the lips, helping to balance them with the rest of the face. To correct a wide lip shape, follow these steps:

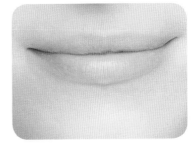

1. Cover the entire lip with your foundation colour.

2. Using a lip pencil, draw a line just inside the lip line on the top and bottom lips.

3. Using the same lip pencil, fill inside the new lip line. Do not use a darker colour, as this will make the lips look fuller.

4. Apply lip colour or gloss to finish the correction.

THIN

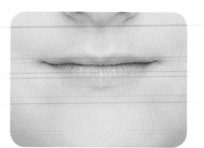

With thin lips, the top and bottom lips are narrow and therefore too small for the face shape. The goal is to increase the fullness of the lips to restore balance. To correct a thin lip shape, follow these steps:

1. Cover the lip area with your foundation colour.

2. With your lip pencil, draw a line just above the lip line on top and bottom.

3. Fill inside of the new lip line. You can choose to use a darker lip pencil colour to create additional fullness.

4. Apply the lip colour of your choice and a gloss at the centre of the lip. The gloss gives a 3-D effect to the lip.

COMBINATION

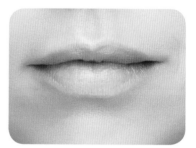

If you have a thin top lip and a full bottom lip (or vice versa), you have a combination lip. The goal is to address the different shapes so they are not only balanced in relation to your face, but also to each other. Follow the steps for correcting thin and wide lips, based on the individual lip shape, to achieve that look.

Avoiding Lip Stains on Your Glass

Would you like to keep your lipstick on your lips and not on the glass of wine you're enjoying? Here's an easy tip: lick the rim of the glass before drinking. Miraculously, your lipstick stays where it should – on your lips!

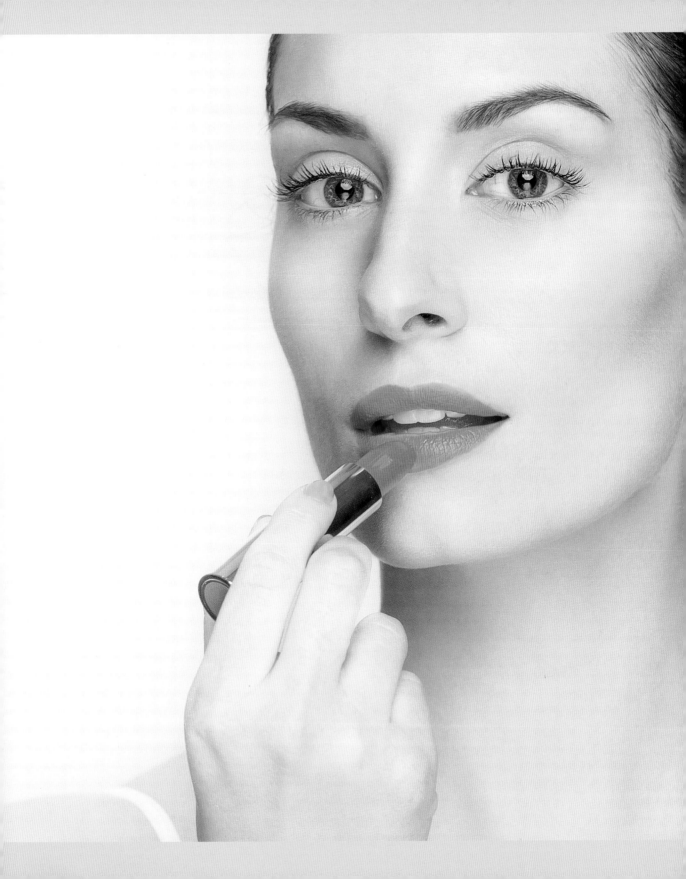

PART 3
BRINGING YOUR LOOK TOGETHER

CHAPTER 13

MAKE-UP CHECKLIST

Before you get into trying some of the sample full make-up applications – the five classic looks – it's time to think about how to document your make-up. After all, you not only want to create a look that's best for you, but also remember it. That's where the make-up checklist comes in.

PROFILE SHEET

I created this profile sheet as a tool for you to better understand your unique face and how your face relates to your make-up choices.

For example, you will often find it difficult to replicate a make-up look you have seen online or in a magazine. That is because the design was on the model in the tutorial, who had her own unique face profile. A good make-up artist has the ability to adapt techniques with each face they encounter. Having a clear understanding of your own face fingerprint will make replicating these looks much easier.

The first part of the profile sheet has you identify your unique facial features, so you know what type of highlighting and contouring you'll need to do to create the most appealing look. In the case of copying a model's look, if you have deep-set eyes and the model doesn't, you have to consider how you apply the same eye shadows in a personally flattering way.

The second half of the profile sheet evaluates your skin type and the basic make-up choices that coordinate with your skin type. This will become your guide for everyday make-up foundation. Keep in mind that skin concerns and colour can change based on time of year – you may have lighter, dryer skin in the winter and darker, breakout-prone skin in the summer. Therefore, a few items on this profile sheet may change throughout the year.

If necessary, go back through the book as you fill out the profile sheet to ensure you're making the most accurate choices.

NAME:_____ AGE:_____

1.	**FACE SHAPE**	Oval	Oblong (Rectangle)	Heart	Diamond	Round	Square

2.	**EYE SHAPE**	Almond	Wide Set	Close Set	Deep Set	Prominent	Small
		Monolid	Hooded	Upturned	Downturned		

3.	**EYE COLOUR**	Blue	Green	Brown	Hazel

4.	**EYEBROWS**	Round	Angled	Soft Angled	Curved	Flat

5.	**NOSE**	Natural	Wide	Thin	Long	Short

6.	**LIPS**	Average	Wide	Thin	Combination

7.	**SKIN TYPE**	Normal	Oily	Dry	Combination	Sensitive

8.	**AREAS OF CONCERN**	Acne	Rosacea	Dark Circles	Dark Spots/ Age Spots	Scars	Redness

9.	**SKIN TONE**	Warm	Cool

10.	**PRIMER**	Clear	Red	Green	Yellow	Purple

11.	**FOUNDATION**	Cream	Liquid	Tinted	Pressed Powder	Mineral

FACE SHEET

Now that you have a better understanding of what works for your face and skin type, you can begin building an individual make-up design.

A handy tool to have as part of your make-up checklist is a face sheet, something you may have seen a make-up artist use at the make-up counter at some point. Basically, you include the following information on a face sheet:

- **Foundation/concealer:** Includes primers, concealers, foundations, or setting powders

- **Corrective make-up:** Includes highlights and contours

- **Eyes:** Includes eye shadows, eyeliners, mascara, or false eyelashes

- **Cheeks:** Includes cheek colours

- **Lips:** Includes lip pencil, lipstick, or lip gloss

To fill out this sheet, use your finger, a brush, or a disposable applicator to apply make-up on the sheet based on what you use to create your look. You can then label the product used in the free space provided. I would suggest applying make-up on the face sheet exactly how you applied it to your face so you more accurately see how the colours looked.

The next page shows you a blank face sheet. If you'd like to see one filled out, check out any of the looks in Chapter 17.

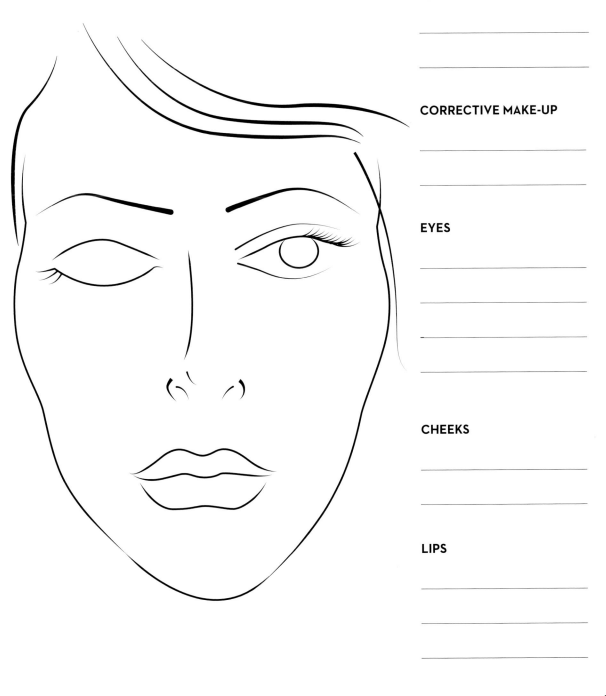

FOUNDATION/CONCEALER

_____

_____

_____

CORRECTIVE MAKE-UP

_____

_____

EYES

_____

_____

_____

_____

CHEEKS

_____

_____

LIPS

_____

_____

_____

CHAPTER 14
FIVE CLASSIC LOOKS

Now that you have the knowledge, the tools, and the tips, let's put a look together! In this chapter, I provide five make-up applications I feel stand the test of time: daytime natural, elegant evening, dramatic evening, metallic smoky eye, and youthful glitter.

Each look includes a completed face sheet and profile sheet for each model, in order to help guide you in mapping out the look for your unique face shape, facial features, and skin type. As you'll see, even a little make-up can make a big impact!

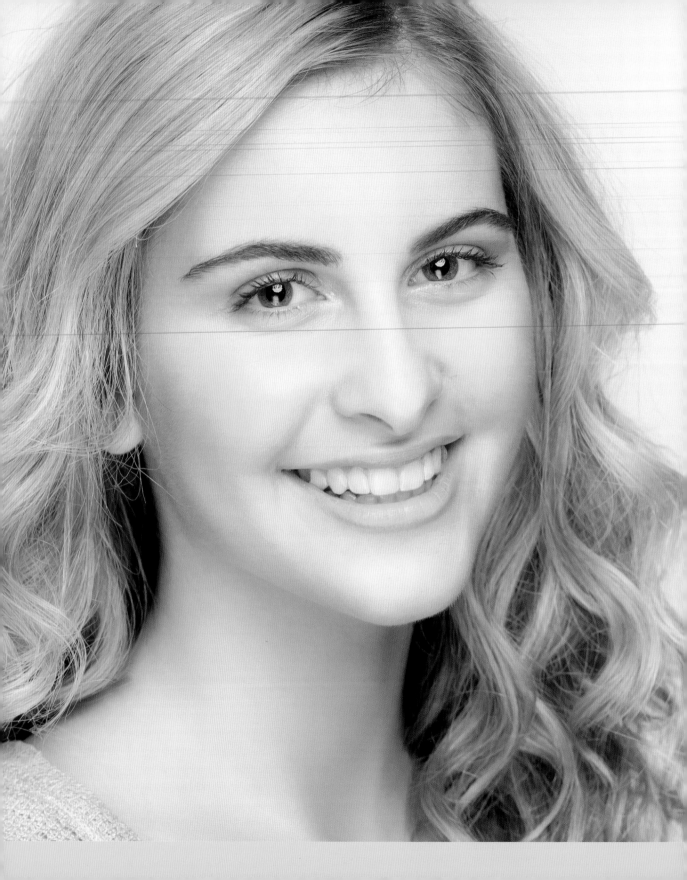

DAYTIME
natural

Make-up doesn't have to be complicated. The key to a daytime look is keeping your make-up light and translucent. A simple eye, a little mascara, and a glossy lip are all you need for a beautifully natural look.

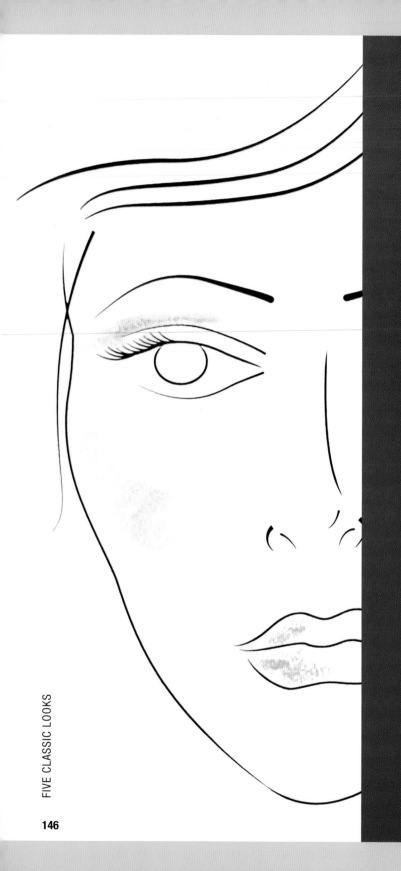

DAYTIME NATURAL
FACE SHEET

FOUNDATION/CONCEALER:
Concealer (half-shade lighter)
Tinted liquid foundation

CORRECTIVE MAKE-UP:
Cream highlight

EYES:
Ivory eye shadow
Taupe eye shadow
Dark brown mascara

CHEEKS:
Peach-pink blusher

LIPS:
Peach-pink jumbo cream
lip pencil
Clear lip gloss

FIVE CLASSIC LOOKS

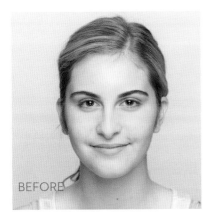

BEFORE

DAYTIME NATURAL
PROFILE SHEET

NAME: Josie

AGE: 16

FACE SHAPE: oval

EYE SHAPE: deep set

EYE COLOUR: green

EYEBROWS: curved

NOSE: natural

LIPS: average

SKIN TYPE: dry

AREAS OF CONCERN: none

SKIN TONE: warm

PRIMER: none

FOUNDATION: liquid

Tools

Disposable latex sponge

Blusher brush

Large eye shadow brush

Medium eye shadow brush

Eyelash curler

Disposable mascara wand

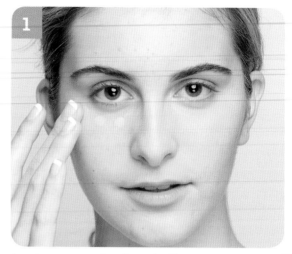

Apply a concealer that's half a shade lighter under the eyes and around the nose and lips, to conceal any redness or trouble spots.

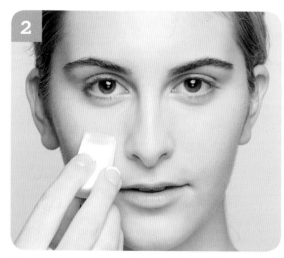

Using a sponge, apply tinted liquid foundation. The tinted moisturizer helps create a sheer, natural look.

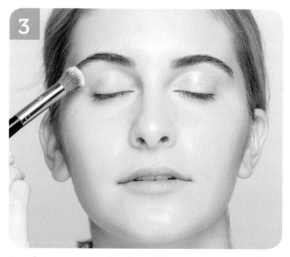

Apply ivory eye shadow all over each eyelid, starting at the brow bone and working your way down to the upper lash line.

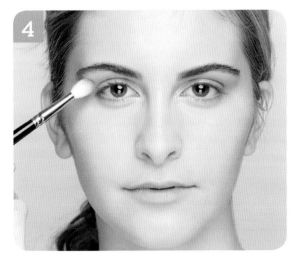

Apply a matte medium taupe eye shadow in each crease.

Eye Shadow for Deep-Set Eyes

Josie has deep-set eyes, so using eye shadow highlight helps bring her eyes forwards. If you have deep-set eyes, you can do the same and use the same shadow under the eye and into the upper cheek to add a highlight. Avoid using dark colours on the eyelids, as that will make your eyes appear they're set back even deeper.

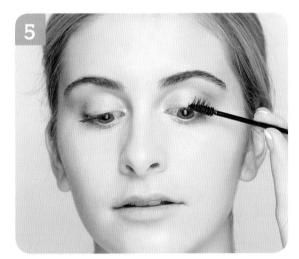

After prepping the eyelashes with an eyelash curler, apply dark brown mascara on the top lashes only.

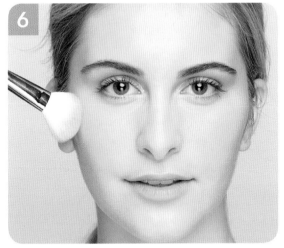

Apply peach-pink cream blusher to the cheeks, making sure you follow the natural cheekbones. Dust a cream highlight onto the cheeks for a bright, dewy look.

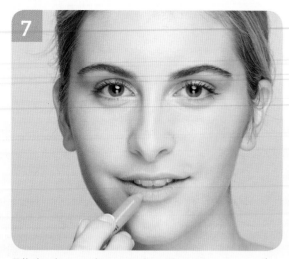

7

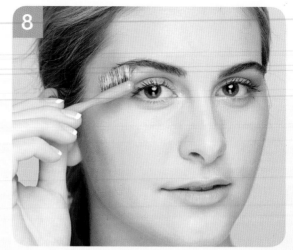

8

Fill the lips with a peach-pink jumbo cream lip pencil to enhance the natural lip colour. You can add a bit of shine to the lips with a clear lip gloss.

Refresh the eyebrows by brushing them with a disposable mascara wand or an eyebrow brush tool.

Creating a Dewy Look

If you want a natural "dewy" look, choose a liquid foundation, cream highlighter, and cream cheek colour. Cream make-up will make your skin look more supple and moisturized than powder. The exception, of course, is if you have oily skin; avoid creams, since they'll be more likely to break out your skin.

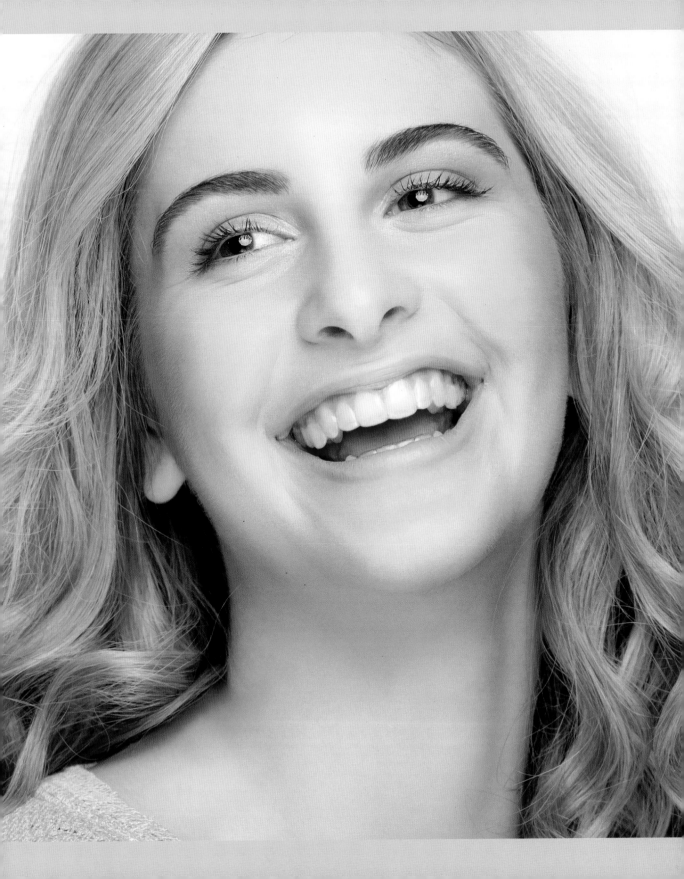

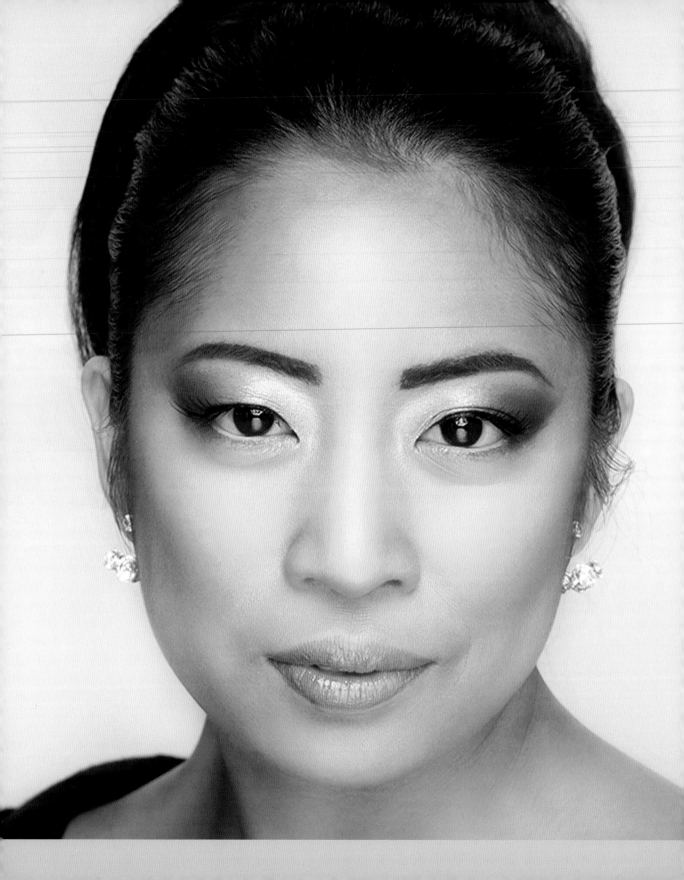

ELEGANT
evening

This full make-up application with a focus on the eye is perfect for special occasions, such as an evening wedding, a glamorous party, or gala event. Because the lighting at a formal evening event tends to be subdued, using a shimmer eye shadow can reflect the lighting in a way that gives you a romantic glow. You can even add some strip eyelashes to ramp up this elegant look.

ELEGANT EVENING

FACE SHEET

FOUNDATION/CONCEALER:
Concealer (half-shade lighter)
Full-coverage liquid foundation

CORRECTIVE MAKE-UP:
Cream highlight
Brown cream eye shadow
Tinted setting powder

EYES:
Black eyebrow pencil
Eye shadow (one shade
lighter than skin tone)
Shimmer taupe eye shadow
Pale yellow shimmer eye
shadow
Dark brown matte eye shadow
Flesh-coloured eye pencil
Black liquid eyeliner
Black mascara

CHEEKS:
Dusty rose blusher

LIPS:
Matte raspberry jumbo lip pencil
Nude lip gloss

ELEGANT EVENING
PROFILE SHEET

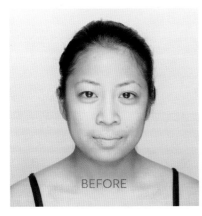

BEFORE

NAME: Arianne

AGE: 23

FACE SHAPE: round

EYE SHAPE: monolid

EYE COLOUR: brown

EYEBROWS: soft angled

NOSE: wide

LIPS: wide

SKIN TYPE: dry and sensitive

AREAS OF CONCERN: none

SKIN TONE: warm

PRIMER: none

FOUNDATION: liquid

Tools

Foundation brush

Powder brush

Blusher brush

Large eye shadow brush

Medium eye shadow brush

Eyelash curler

False strip eyelashes, eyelash glue, and cosmetic scissors (optional)

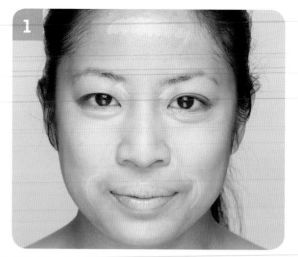

Apply concealer that's half a shade lighter under the eyes, around the nose, on the "brackets" around the lips, on the forehead, and on the chin.

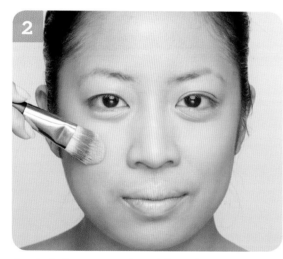

Apply full-coverage liquid foundation.

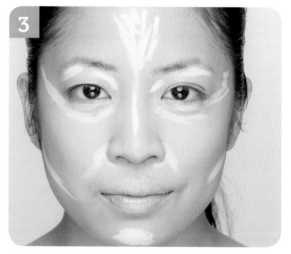

Apply cream highlight under the cheeks, along the nose and middle of the forehead, around the nose, under the eyes and eyebrows, and on the chin.

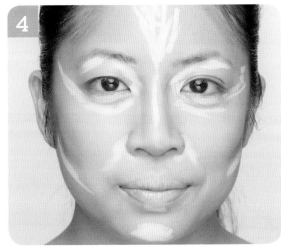

Apply brown eye shadow contour along the cheekbones, sides of the nose, tip of the nose, along the jawline, and above the hairline at the temple.

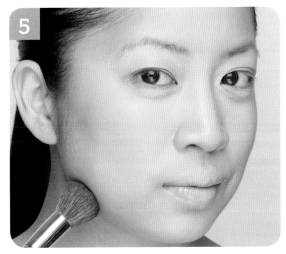

Blend the highlight and contour by brushing on tinted setting powder.

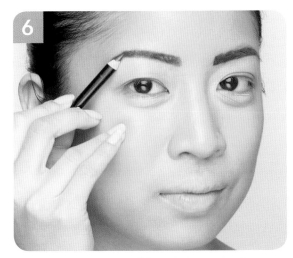

Use a black pencil to fill and shape the brows. This will create dynamic, soft-angled brows.

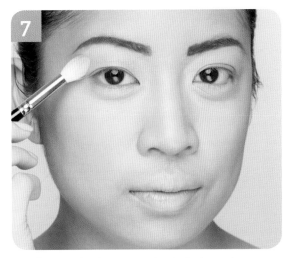

Apply eye shadow one shade lighter than your natural skin tone under the brow bones and down into the corner of the eyes.

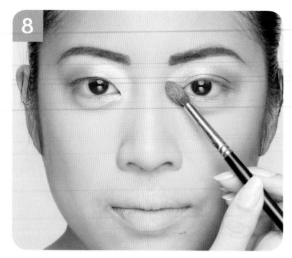

Apply shimmer taupe eye shadow from the tear ducts over the eyelids. Open your eyes and reapply. Apply pale yellow shimmer eye shadow from the inside corner of the eye, stopping just before the centre.

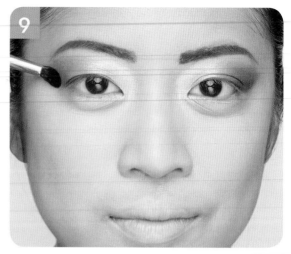

Apply dark brown matte shadow to the outer corners of the eyelids.

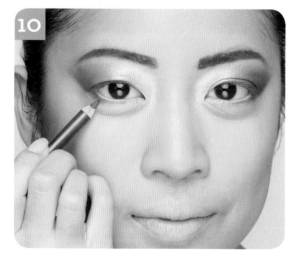

Apply a flesh-coloured pencil followed by a brown pencil onto the water line to give the illusion of wider eyes.

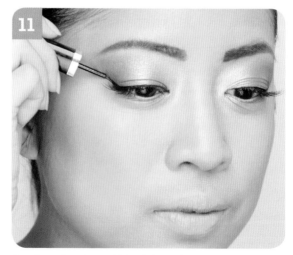

Apply a thin line of black liquid eyeliner, starting in the corner of each eye and following the natural lash line around; end with a thin wing tip.

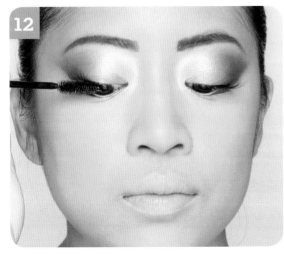

After curling the eyelashes, apply black mascara to the top lashes.

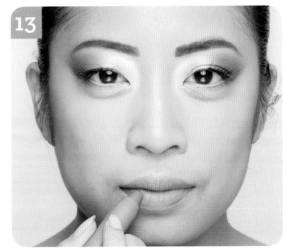

Apply dusty rose blusher to the cheeks. Fill and line the lips with a matte raspberry jumbo lip pencil. Dab lip gloss (either nude or a shade similar to the lip colour) onto the centre of the lips for highlight.

Optional Strip Lash

Before putting on mascara, add half a false strip eyelash to the corner of the eyes to fill out your lashes. Simply cut a strip lash in half and use the fuller half on the upper lash line.

Making Your Eyes Appear Larger

To make your eyes appear larger, apply a white liner on the lower water line. Next, directly underneath the white line, apply a brown or black eyeliner. This will give the illusion of a larger eye.

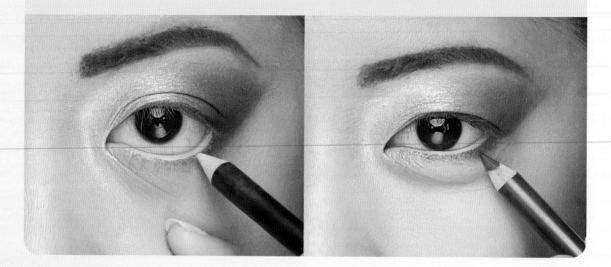

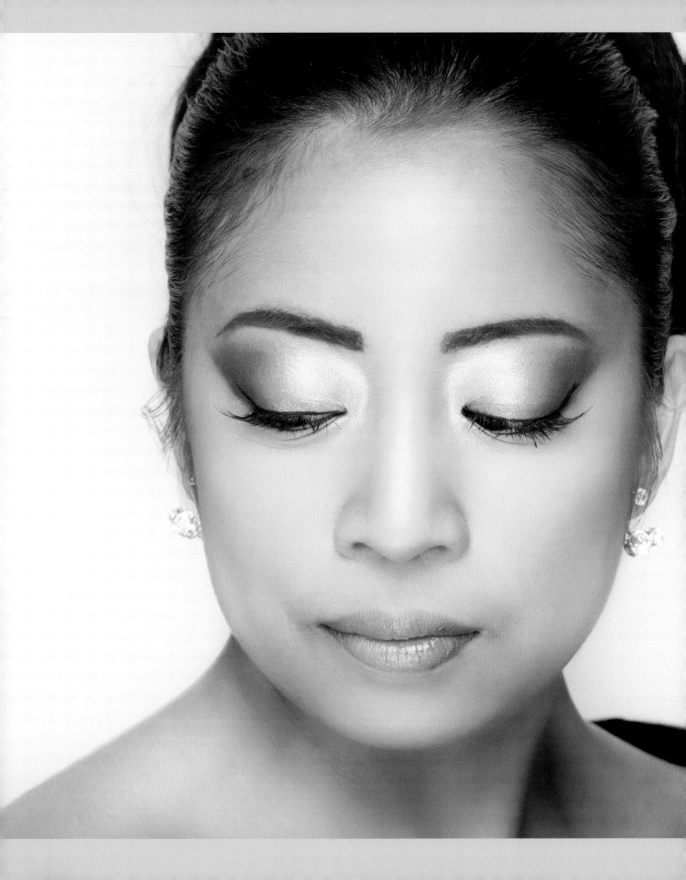

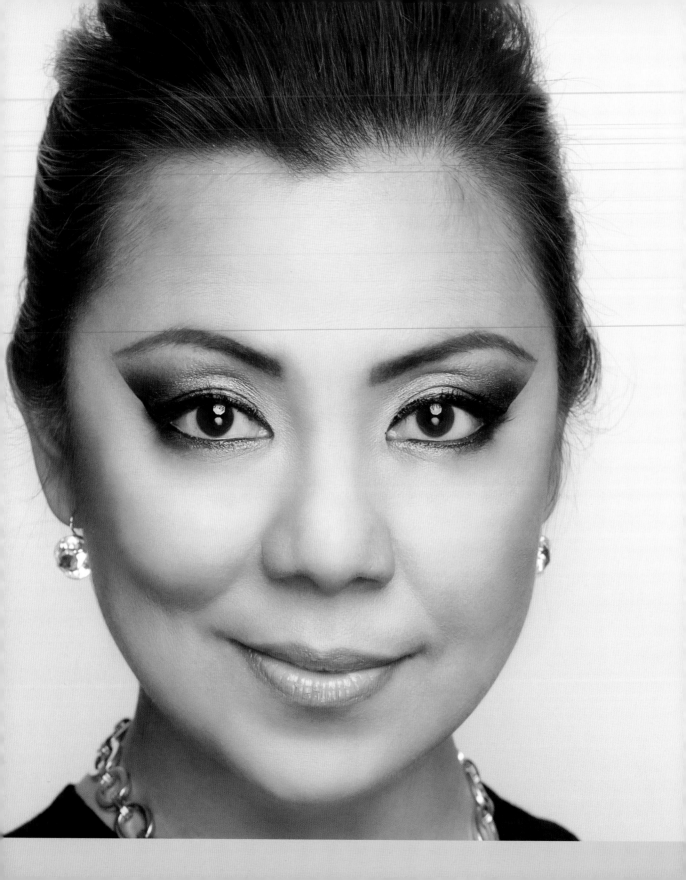

DRAMATIC
evening

When you are going out to a club, for a night out with the girls, or anywhere you can let loose, you have a chance to go really bold with your make-up! As for the elegant evening make-up, the lighting in most night-time venues is darker, making it a prime opportunity to create drama with your look. For this dramatic look, you'll make the eyes your showy statement piece.

DRAMATIC EVENING
FACE SHEET

FOUNDATION/CONCEALER:
Concealer
Full-coverage cream foundation

CORRECTIVE MAKE-UP:
Cream highlight pencil

EYES:
Dark brown eyebrow pencil
Pale gold shimmer eye shadow
Bronze shimmer eye shadow
Teal shimmer eye shadow
Midnight blue shimmer eye shadow
Black liquid eyeliner
Black mascara

CHEEKS:
Dusty rose blusher

LIPS:
Flesh-coloured lip pencil
Flesh-coloured lip gloss

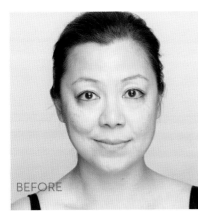

BEFORE

DRAMATIC EVENING
PROFILE SHEET

NAME: *Nathalie*

AGE: *39*

FACE SHAPE: *round*

EYE SHAPE: *monolid*

EYE COLOUR: *brown*

EYEBROWS: *soft angled*

NOSE: *wide*

LIPS: *wide*

SKIN TYPE: *oily*

AREAS OF CONCERN: *dark circles*

SKIN TONE: *warm*

PRIMER: *clear*

FOUNDATION: *cream*

Tools

Disposable latex sponge

Blusher brush

Large eye shadow brush

Medium eye shadow brush

Sticky tape

Index card

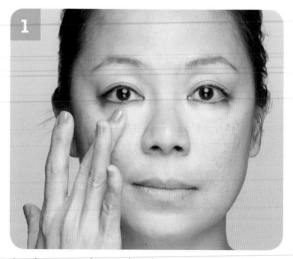

1

Apply concealer under the eyes, around the nose, and wherever else you have redness.

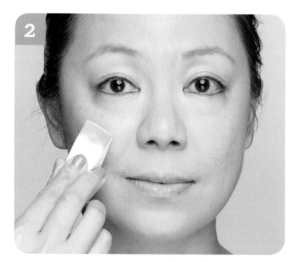

2

Apply full-coverage cream foundation.

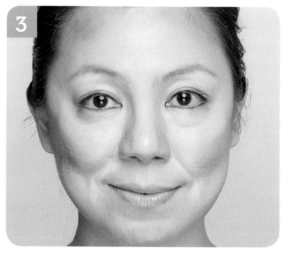

3

Apply highlight and contour to the cheeks, nose, jawline, and forehead. Blend highlight and contour into the foundation with a damp sponge.

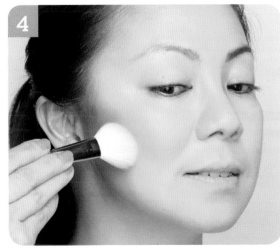

Brush a soft dusty rose blusher between highlight and contour, following the natural line of the cheeks.

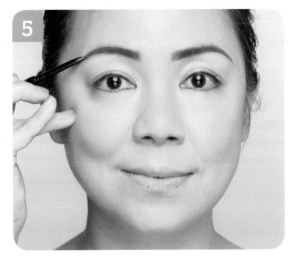

With a dark brown pencil, start filling in the eyebrows from the inside corner of the eye, creating "hair strokes" straight up and angled towards the natural brow shape. The brows should be slightly fuller near the nose and thinner from the arch to the end of the brow.

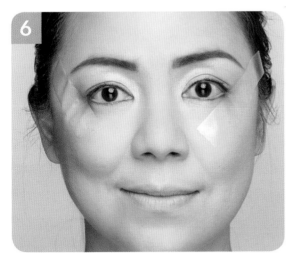

Place sticky tape along the outside of the eyes, starting at the outside corner and angling to the end of the eyebrows; this will help you with placement. Apply pale gold shimmer eye shadow from the corner of each eye and follow up across the entire eyebrow, ending at the brow bone to create a crease.

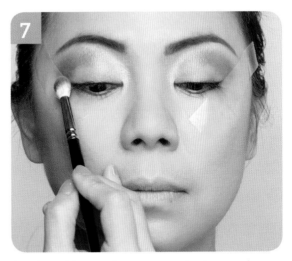

Apply a shimmer bronze eye shadow under the gold highlight (on the upper crease) on each eye.

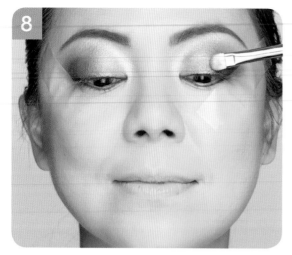

Apply teal shimmer eye shadow on the lash lines and into the crease of each eyelid.

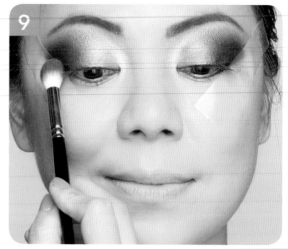

Apply midnight blue shimmer shadow at the end of the lash line, swooping up along the edge to create a smoky eye.

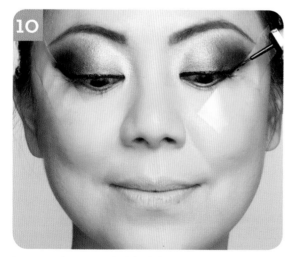

Line each eye with black liquid eyeliner by following the lash line and travelling up the side of the tape. Apply black eyeliner on the lower water lines for a dramatic look. When finished, gently remove the tape.

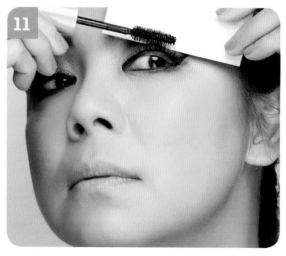

Load up the eyelashes with an intense black mascara. You can place an index card in front of the eyelids to avoid creating streaks.

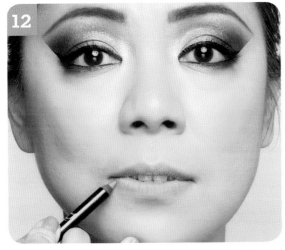

Use a flesh-coloured lip pencil to line and fill in the lips.

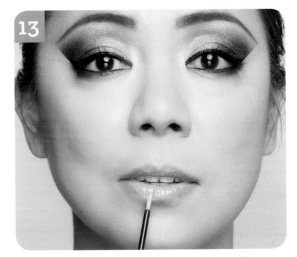

Apply flesh-coloured lip gloss on top of the lip pencil.

The Sticky Tape Method

Here's a tip for a flawless eye shadow application:

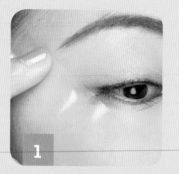

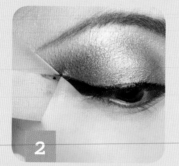

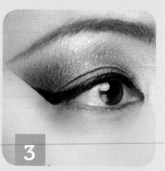

1 Place a piece of sticky tape at an angle from the outside corner of the eye to the end of the eyebrow, before you apply your eye shadows.

2 When you have finished, carefully remove the tape.

3 As you can see, you're left with a clean shadow line. People will think you've had your make-up done by a professional!

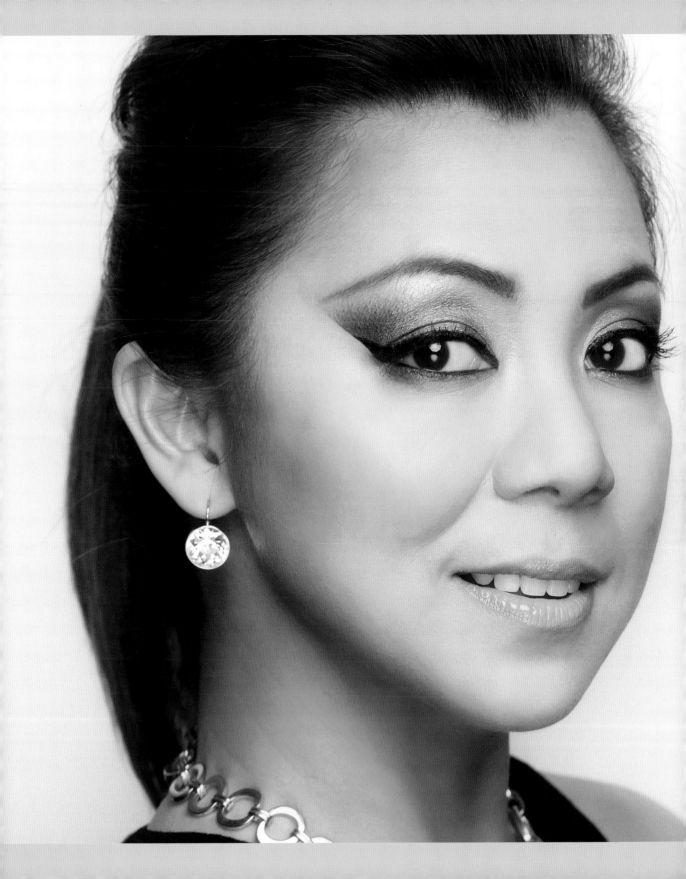

METALLIC
smoky eye

The typical smoky eye is created by blending greys and blacks onto the eyelid. This look uses a metallic silver shadow in place of the grey, giving a contemporary twist to the traditional smoky eye. Metallic looks like this are especially fabulous for darker skin tones.

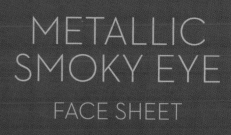

METALLIC
SMOKY EYE
FACE SHEET

FOUNDATION/CONCEALER:
Orange-brown cream primer
Full-coverage liquid foundation

CORRECTIVE MAKE-UP:
Cream highlight
Brown cream contour
Tinted setting powder

EYES:
Black eyeliner pencil
Highlight cream eye shadow
White eye shadow
Gunmetal metallic eye shadow
Black eye shadow
Silver metallic liquid eye
shadow
Black mascara

CHEEKS:
Orange cream blusher

LIPS:
Flesh-coloured lip pencil
Apricot lip gloss

METALLIC SMOKY EYE
PROFILE SHEET

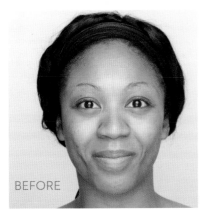

BEFORE

NAME: Ashley

AGE: 32

FACE SHAPE: diamond

EYE SHAPE: wide set and monolid

EYE COLOUR: brown

EYEBROWS: soft angled

NOSE: wide

LIPS: wide

SKIN TYPE: combination

AREAS OF CONCERN: dark spots

SKIN TONE: cool

PRIMER: orange

FOUNDATION: liquid

Tools

Medium eye shadow brush

Concealer brush

Beauty sponge

Powder brush

Large eye shadow brush

Angle brush

Dual-fibre brush

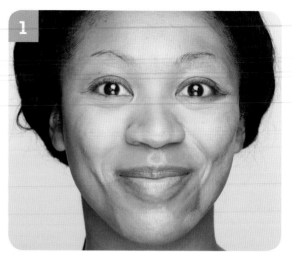

Apply orange-brown cream primer under the eyes and brow bones, around the nose, on the chin, and on any other trouble spots.

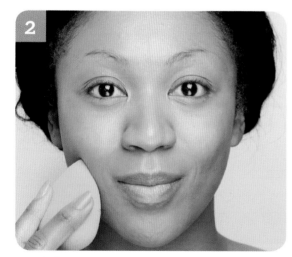

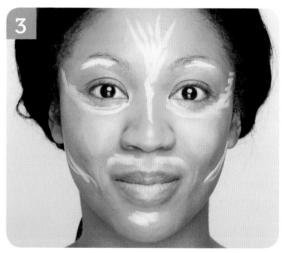

Apply full-coverage liquid foundation.

Apply cream highlight under the brow bones, between the eyebrows, and up the forehead. Continue application down the centre of the nose, under the eyelids to the hairline, above the lips, under the hollows of the cheeks, and on the middle of the chin.

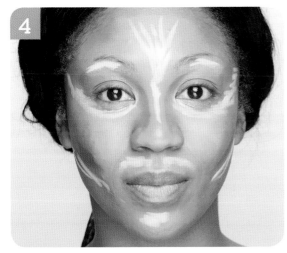

Apply brown cream contour to the hollows of the cheeks, under the chin, above the highlight on the temples, and from along the sides of the nose to the corners of the eyes.

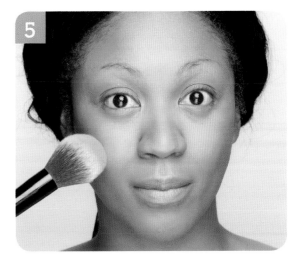

Use tinted setting powder to blend the contour and highlight.

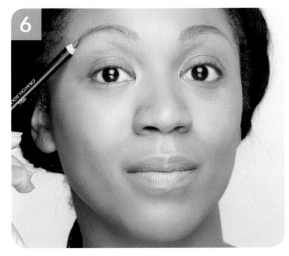

Use black eyeliner to create curved eyebrows.

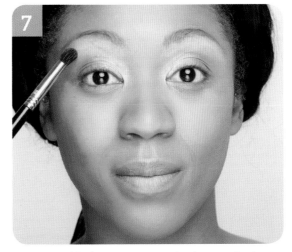

Apply highlight cream eye shadow to the brow bones and white eye shadow in the centre of the nose contour. Then place white eye shadow in the corners of the eyes, brushing it up and onto the brow bones.

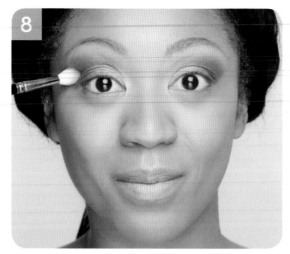

Apply gunmetal metallic eye shadow for contour in the crease, making sure to blend it to the outer edges of the lids.

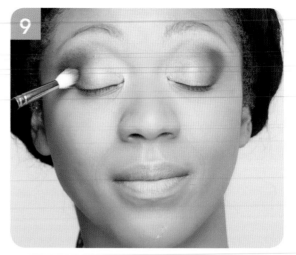

Apply black eye shadow to the corners of each eye and blend to the crease, making sure to blend in circular motions. This creates the smoky-eye effect.

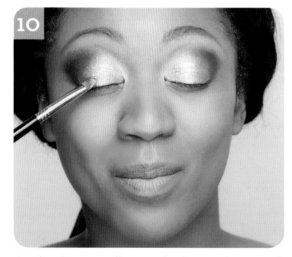

Apply silver metallic eye shadow to the rest of the eyelids.

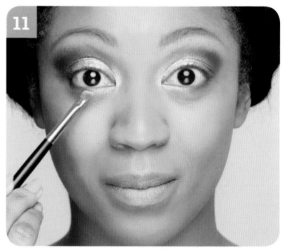

Using black eye shadow, create a soft, smoky line starting at the outside corner of the lower lash line and moving to the middle of the eye. Brush slowly back and forth to blend. Apply silver metallic eye shadow from the tear duct to the middle of the lower lid, connecting it to the black shadow. Swipe back and forth to diffuse and blend the colours.

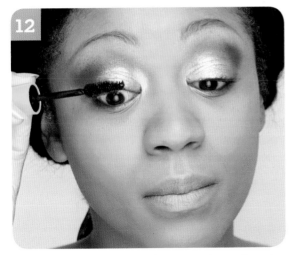

Apply black eyeliner to the water line of each eye. Finish the eyes by applying black mascara.

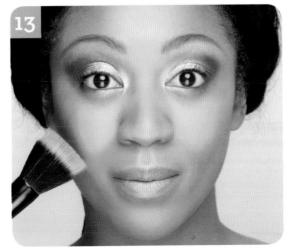

Apply orange blush to the apples of the cheeks.

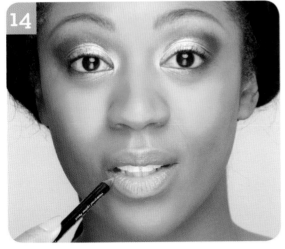

Line and fill the lips with flesh-coloured lip pencil.

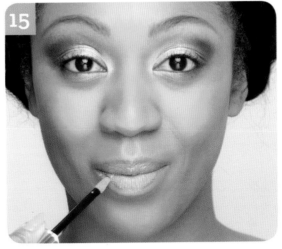

Finish the lips by applying apricot lip gloss.

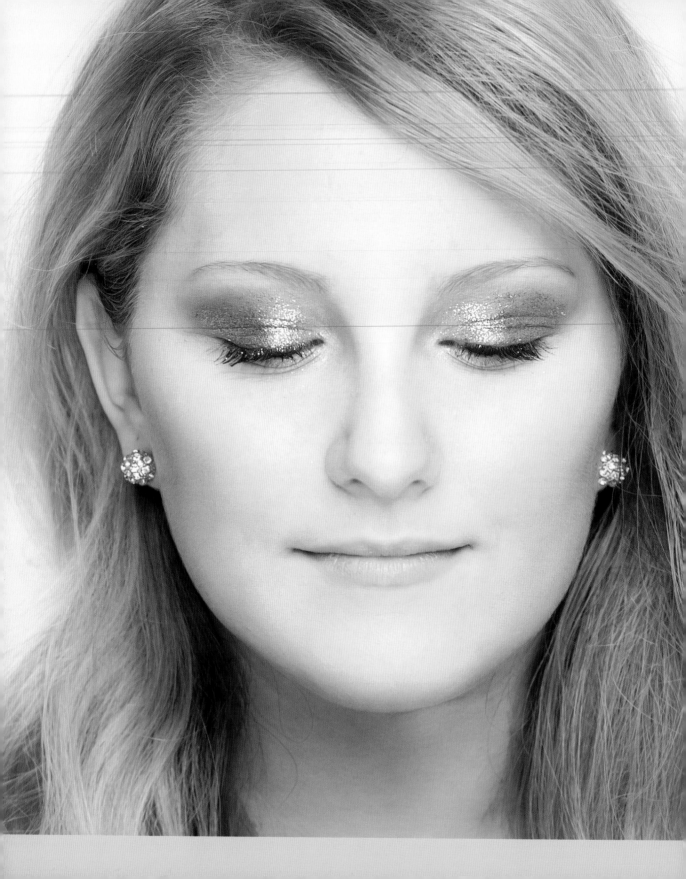

YOUTHFUL
glitter

Cosmetic glitter is a great makeup tool for creating a fun and sassy look. It is nontoxic and comes in many different fun shades. While this strong of a glitter look should be left to the very young, older women can certainly include elements for an evening look. Because glitter should be the leading player in this youthful look, keep your cheeks and lips neutral!

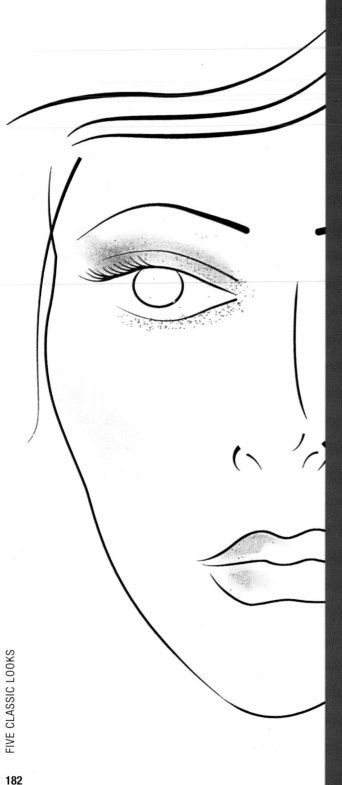

YOUTHFUL GLITTER
FACE SHEET

FOUNDATION/CONCEALER:

Cream concealer

Moisture tint foundation

CORRECTIVE MAKE-UP:

Powder highlight

EYES:

Taupe eye shadow

Emerald green shimmer eye shadow

Frosty white eye shadow

Black mascara

Jade green cosmetic glitter

CHEEKS:

Dusty rose powder blusher

LIPS:

Fleshy pink matte lip pencil

YOUTHFUL GLITTER
PROFILE SHEET

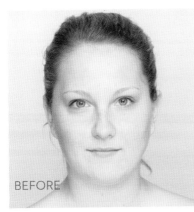

BEFORE

NAME: Brooke

AGE: 19

FACE SHAPE: square

EYE SHAPE: downturned

EYE COLOUR: blue-green

EYEBROWS: curved

NOSE: thin

LIPS: combination

SKIN TYPE: dry

AREAS OF CONCERN: none

SKIN TONE: cool

PRIMER: none

FOUNDATION: liquid

Tools

Blusher brush

Angle brush

Large eye shadow brush

Medium eye shadow brush

Cotton bud

Tissues

Cosmetic glue (optional)

Sticky tape

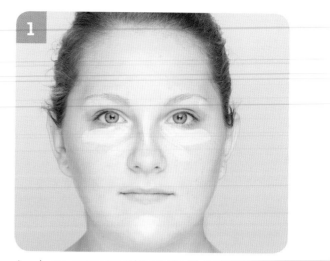

Apply cream concealer under the eyes, around the nose, and on the chin.

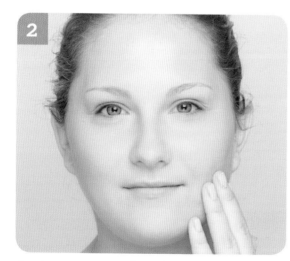

Apply moisture tint foundation all over the face, using the fingers.

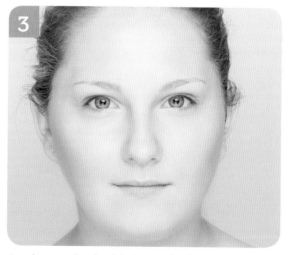

Apply powder highlight on the brow bones, cheekbones, and nose.

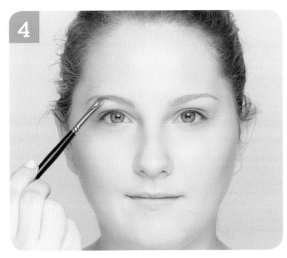

Apply taupe eye shadow to the eyebrows to reshape them.

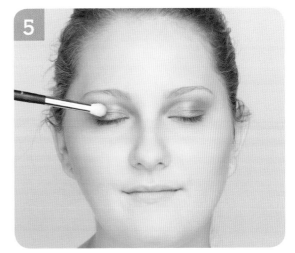

Apply emerald green shimmer eye shadow on the lid up to just above the crease. This creates a background colour to the glitter, particularly for hooded eyes.

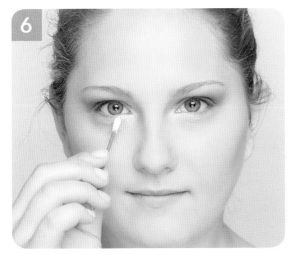

With a cotton bud, apply frosty white eye shadow at the corner of the eyes and lightly under the bottom lash lines.

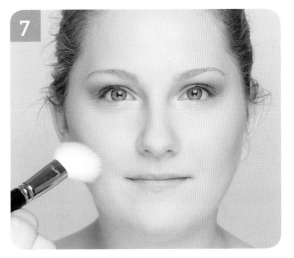

Brush on dusty rose blusher, blending it into the apples of the cheeks.

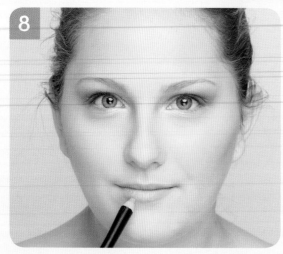

8

Apply fleshy pink matte lip pencil just above the natural lip line to create fuller lips.

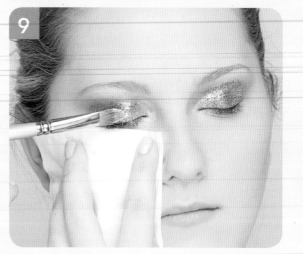

9

For each eye, place a tissue under the eyelash, close the eye, and gently press jade green cosmetic glitter onto the eyelid with a brush. Cosmetic glitter glue can be used if necessary to secure the glitter.

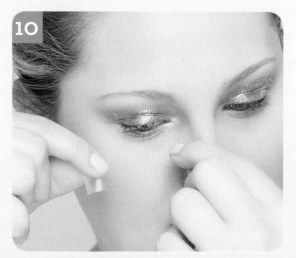

10

Glitter Warning

When using cosmetic glitter, less is more. It is easy to make the glitter look messy by applying too much.

Use a piece of sticky tape to remove any glitter that has fallen onto the cheeks or elsewhere on the face. Apply several coats of black mascara.

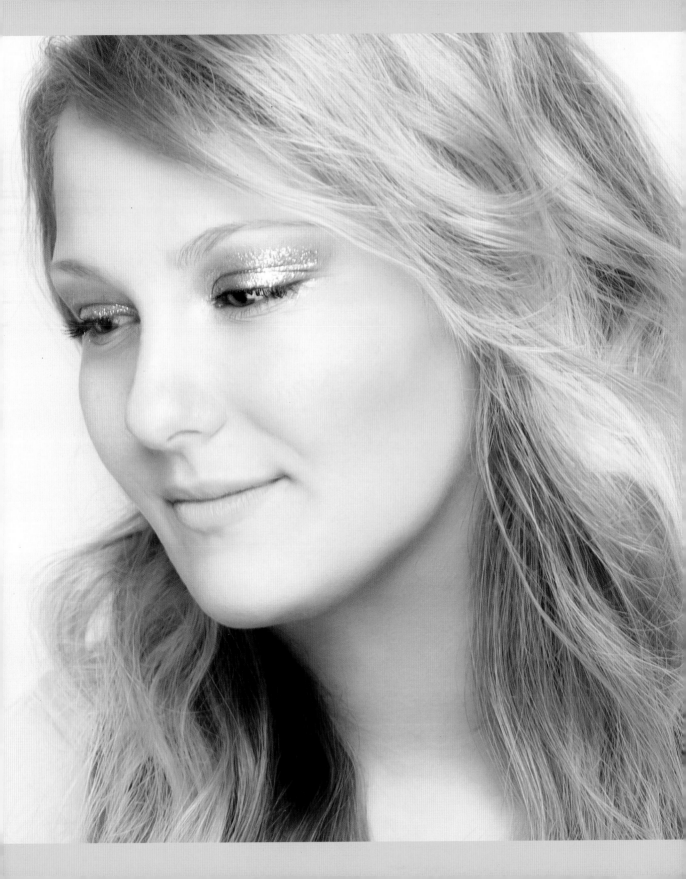

GLOSSARY

airbrushing   A combination of a concentrated pigment with a flow of air. It essentially mists the make-up onto your skin, creating a natural silkscreen effect.

beauty sponge   A sponge applicator without edges. You can use a beauty sponge to blend make-up after applying it with your fingers or a make-up brush.

bridge   The cartilage running down the centre of the nose.

bronzer   A product used to imitate a suntan. It is considered a natural look and is often used for everyday wear. It highlights your cheekbones and contours your face. Bronzer is an easy way to enhance colour and provide shimmer to your skin tone.

chemical exfoliant   A product that utilizes chemicals such as hydroxy acids (lactic acid, salicylic acid, and glycolic acid), retinol (vitamin A), or enzymes (papain, bromelain, and protease enzymes from *Bacillus* microbes) to create cell turnover in the epidermis. This stimulates the formation of normal, healthy skin.

complementary colours   Colours that are opposite each other on the colour wheel. When combined in the right proportions, they create white or black. Complementary colours can help you choose which shades work best for everything from your skin's undertone to your eyes, lips, and nails.

concealer   A flesh-toned cosmetic product used to cover dark circles, discolouration, age spots, and blemishes. It is similar to foundation, but thicker.

contour   Giving shape to an area of your face and enhancing your facial structure through the use of make-up. Contour uses a powder or cream make-up product typically one to two shades darker than your skin colour.

corrective make-up   Using highlight (light) and contour (dark/shadow) to change the shape of your face. Corrective make-up highlights features you find attractive and disguises your less flattering features.

emphasis   The areas to which you want to draw attention. Make-up uses colour as emphasis to direct attention to different parts of your face, such as your lips or your eyes.

exfoliant   Products designed to remove dead cells from the surface of your skin. *See also* mechanical exfoliant *and* chemical exfoliant.

eyelash curler   A tool used to curl your eyelashes prior to applying mascara or false eyelashes.

eyelash primer   A cosmetic that coats your eyelashes, protecting them against damage from mascara. Primers provide moisture to dry lashes and allow your mascara to go on evenly.

face sheet   A document used to record what cosmetics you used to achieve a certain look and where you placed those products on your face. A face sheet is typically broken into three sections: eyes, cheeks, and lips.

ferrule   The metal portion of a make-up brush that holds the bristles in place.

foundation   Skin-coloured make-up used to even out your skin tone, cover flaws, and sometimes change the colour of your face.

highlight   The process of lightening an area to bring it forwards or make it more prominent. Highlight uses powder or cream make-up products one to two shades lighter than your skin colour.

kabuki brush   A brush specially made for the application of mineral make-up. The design of the brush, with its short handle and dense bristles, assists in a heavier application necessary for this make-up.

mechanical exfoliant   A product that employs the use of either a tool (for example, a brush or sponge) or substrate (for example, rice bran, date seed powder, or oatmeal) to stimulate cell turnover. Depending on the amount of friction and the nature of abrasive used, a mechanical exfoliant loosens and reduces the outer layer of skin cells.

mineral make-up   A make-up comprising 100 per cent minerals (such as titanium dioxide, zinc oxide, mica, and iron oxide), which is free from organic dyes, preservatives, and fragrance. Many ancient cultures used ground-up natural minerals as a means of applying colour to the skin for decoration, camouflage, and war paint.

monolid   An eye shape in which there is little to no crease in the eyelid and no brow bone. With a monolid, there is a fairly flat surface between your eyelid and your eyebrow.

pH   A measurement of acidity or alkalinity. The pH of healthy skin is 4.5 to 5.5.

primary colours   Refers to a group of colours that can be mixed together to make all other colours. Red, yellow, and blue are the primary colours.

primer   A cream or lotion applied to improve the coverage and duration of your make-up. A primer is applied before a concealer. *See also* tinted primer.

salicylic acid   A beta-hydroxy acid used to treat acne.

secondary colours   A combination of two or more primary colours. Orange, green, and violet are secondary colours.

setting powder   A type of powder used for reducing oil on your face, setting cream foundation, and blending contour.

shimmer   A type of eye shadow that has light-reflecting materials included. Shimmer gives depth and interest to the many shades of eye shadow available.

smoky eye   A dramatic style of eye make-up that gives your eyes a dark, smoky appearance. Its popularity began in the 1920s. The typical smoky eye uses black and grey eye shadows and black liner applied in a circular pattern around the eyes.

SPF   The acronym for sun protection factor, referring to the ability of a sunscreen to block ultraviolet rays. An SPF rating is listed on many moisturizers and foundations that include sunscreen to protect your skin.

T-zone   Where your skin tends to become the most oily. To find your T-zone, draw an imaginary line across your forehead and another line from your nose to your chin.

tattoo cover   A very thick cosmetic product with a matte finish that's used to cover up the dark and multicoloured ink of a tattoo.

tertiary colours   A combination of a primary and secondary colour. Red-orange, red-violet, yellow-orange, yellow-green, blue-violet, and blue-green are tertiary colours.

tinted primer   A cream or lotion available in red, green, yellow, or violet. It is used to neutralize problem areas on the skin, such as rosacea, acne, dark circles, and any other skin discolourations.

toner   A skin care product that's balanced to return skin to its proper pH. Additionally, toners remove excess debris and reduce pore size.

UV rays   Refers to ultraviolet radiation, the energy radiating from the sun. Products such as sunscreen, some moisturizers, and foundations display a sun protection factor to show how they protect your skin from these harmful rays.

INDEX